Working for Equality in Health

Widening social inequalities in Britain are reflected in uneven patterns of health within and between populations. Among professional health workers there is a developing awareness of the significance of tackling inequality in order to secure better health. In *Working for Equality in Health*, the contributors, who include health activists, service users and carers, politicians and researchers as well as health and social care professionals, not only detail the interrelationships and processes by which health inequalities are maintained, but present analyses – refined through experience – of strategies to combat them. They describe their attempts in practice to counteract the impact on people's health of the complex interaction of inequalities based on class, relative poverty, 'race', gender, age, disability and sexual orientation.

Working for Equality in Health brings to bear the understanding of a unique combination of practitioners and activists on a key issue for health experience, policy and practice. Common themes and common obstacles become apparent: the need for ever better understandings of the interactive effects of social disadvantage; the damage wrought to people's health by inegalitarian economic, social and health policies and the benefits of alliances between health professionals and other health workers built upon a strategic commitment to combat social and health inequalities.

Paul Bywaters is a Principal Lecturer in the School of Health and Social Sciences at Coventry University. **Eileen McLeod** is a Senior Lecturer in Applied Social Studies at the University of Warwick.

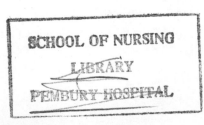

The State of Welfare
Edited by Mary Langan

Nearly half a century after its post-war consolidation, the British welfare state is once again at the centre of political controversy. After a decade in which the role of the state in the provision of welfare was steadily reduced in favour of the private, voluntary and informal sectors, with relatively little public debate or resistance, the further extension of the new mixed economy of welfare in the spheres of health and education became a major political issue in the early 1990s. At the same time the impact of deepening recession has begun to expose some of the deficiencies of market forces in areas such as housing and income maintenance, where their role had expanded dramatically during the 1980s. *The State of Welfare* provides a forum for continuing the debate about the services we need in the 1990s.

Titles of related interest also in *The State of Welfare* series

The Dynamics of British Health Policy
Stephen Harrison, David Hunter and Christopher Pollitt

Radical Social Work Today
Edited by Mary Langan and Phil Lee

Taking Child Abuse Seriously
The Violence Against Children Study Group

Ideologies of Welfare: From Dreams to Disillusion
John Clarke, Allan Cochrane and Carol Smart

Women, Oppression and Social Work
Edited by Mary Langan and Lesley Day

Managing Poverty: The Limits of Social Assistance
Carol Walker

The Eclipse of Council Housing
Ian Cole and Robert Furbey

Towards a Post-Fordist Welfare State?
Roger Burrows and Brian Loader

Working with Men: Feminism and Social Work
Edited by Kate Cavanagh and Viviene E. Cree

Social Theory, Social Change and Social Work
Edited by Nigel Paton

Working for Equality in Health

Edited by Paul Bywaters and
Eileen McLeod

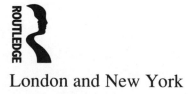

London and New York

First published 1996
by Routledge
11 New Fetter Lane, London EC4P 4EE

Simultaneously published in the USA and Canada
by Routledge
29 West 35th Street, New York, NY 10001

Routledge is an International Thomson Publishing company

Typeset in Times by
Ponting–Green Publishing Services, Chesham, Bucks
Printed and bound in Great Britain by
TJ Press Ltd, Padstow, Cornwall

British Library Cataloguing in Publication Data
A catalogue record for this book is available from the
British Library

Library of Congress Cataloguing in Publication Data
Working for equality in health / edited by Paul Bywaters and
Eileen McLeod
p.   cm.– (The state of welfare)
Includes bibliographical references and index.
1. Poor – Medical care – Great Britain.   2. Socially
handicapped – Medical care – Great Britain.
3.   Discrimination in medical care – Great Britain.
4.   Health services accessibility – Great Britain.
5.   Equality – Great Britain.   6.   Right to health care
– Great Britain.   7.   Medical social work – Great Britain.
I. Bywaters, Paul, 1949–   II. McLeod, Eileen.
III. Series.
RA418.5P6W67   1996
362.1'0941–dc20 95–25987

ISBN   0–415–12465–4 (hbk)
ISBN   0–415–12466–2 (pbk)

To Anna, Dominic, Emma, Michael, Rosie and Sara

Contents

Figures and tables

FIGURES

TABLES

Contributors

Jo Aldridge   Research Officer, Young Carers Research Group, Department of Social Sciences, Loughborough University.

Saul Becker   Director of Studies for the Interdisciplinary Programme in Policy Organization and Change in Professional Care; Director, Young Carers Research Group, Department of Social Studies, Loughborough University.

Clare Blackburn   Research Fellow, Department of Applied Social Studies, University of Warwick.

Paul Bywaters   Principal Lecturer in Social Work, School of Health and Social Sciences, Coventry University.

Mick Carpenter   Senior Lecturer, Department of Applied Social Studies, University of Warwick; Official Historian of COHSE; Academic Adviser to the creation of UNISON.

Jenny Douglas   Director of Health Promotion, Sandwell, West Midlands.

Clare Evans   Convenor, Wiltshire Community Care User Involvement Network, known as Wiltshire Users Network.

Hilary Graham   Professor of Applied Social Studies, Department of Applied Social Studies, University of Warwick.

Eileen McLeod   Senior Lecturer, Department of Applied Social Studies, University of Warwick.

Desmond O'Neill   Consultant Geriatrician, Age Related Health Care, Meath Hospital, Dublin.

Simon Sedgwick-Jell   Ex-leader, Cambridge City Council.

Nick Spencer   Professor of Community Child Health, School of Postgraduate Medical Education and Department of Applied Social Studies, University of Warwick; Consultant Community Paediatrician, Coventry Health Care NHS Trust.

Simon Watney   Director of the Red Hot AIDS Charitable Trust.

Rosie Weaver   Locality Resource Manager, Sparkbrook, Southern Birmingham Community NHS Trust.

Series editor's preface

In the 1990s the perception of a crisis of welfare systems has become universal across the Western world. The coincidence of global economic slump and the ending of the Cold War has intensified pressures to reduce welfare spending at the same time that Western governments, traditional social institutions and political parties all face unprecedented problems of legitimacy. Given the importance of welfare policies in securing popular consent for existing regimes and in maintaining social stability, welfare budgets have in general proved remarkably resilient even in face of governments proclaiming the principles of austerity and self-reliance.

Yet the crisis of welfare has led to measures of reform and retrenchment which have provoked often bitter controversy in virtually every sphere, from hospitals and schools to social security benefits and personal social services. What is striking is the crumbling of the old structures and policies before any clear alternative has emerged. The general impression is one of exhaustion and confusion. There is a widespread sense that everything has been tried and has failed and that nobody is very clear about how to advance into an increasingly bleak future.

On both sides of the Atlantic, the agenda of free market anti-statism has provided the cutting edge for measures of privitization. The result has been a substantial shift in the 'mixed economy' of welfare towards a more market-orientated approach. But it has not taken long for the defects of the market as a mechanism for social regulation to become apparent. Yet now that the inadequacy of the market in providing equitable or even efficient welfare services is exposed, where else is there to turn?

The State of Welfare series aims to provide a critical assessment of the policy implications of some of the wide social and economic changes of the 1990s. Globalization, the emergence of post-industrial society, the transformation of work, demographic shifts and changes in gender roles and family structures all have major consequences for the patterns of welfare provision established half a century ago.

The demands of women and minority ethnic groups, as well as the voices of younger, older and disabled people and the influence of social movements concerned with issues of sexuality, gender and the environment must all be taken into account in the construction of a social policy for the new millennium.

Mary Langan
March 1995

Acknowledgements

We would like to acknowledge our debt to many people. First, we should like to acknowledge the commitment, hard work and good humour of our co-contributors. We are also grateful to Mandy Coult and Jane Lissaman for their excellent work in the typing and preparation of the manuscript and for the exceptional willingness and generosity with which they tackled the many demands of the task. We would also like to thank the Universities of Coventry and Warwick for periods of study leave and other support which enabled this book to get under way. Mary Langan, the series editor, has been helpful at every stage in the process.

Finally we should like to thank Racheal Hards, Olwen Haslam, Anna McLeod and Alison Powell and our hard-pressed working colleagues for their helpful criticisms, encouragement and support.

Part I

Face to face care

Chapter 1

Introduction

Paul Bywaters and Eileen McLeod

There is substantial and mounting evidence that social inequalities profoundly undermine health. There are also strong indications that social inequalities have been widening in Britain in recent years and that this is reflected in worsening inequalities in health: in more widespread, unnecessary, unjust human suffering. Tackling the causes and consequences of these trends is of central importance to a growing number of unpaid and paid health workers. The contributors to this book are all engaged in such work. Here they distil the lessons from their efforts and make proposals for action to secure greater equality in health.

THE RELATIONSHIP BETWEEN SOCIAL INEQUALITIES AND HEALTH INEQUALITIES

Across the past two decades health workers, researchers and lay health activists have been opening up understanding of the relationships between social and health inequalities in Britain. Pioneering epidemiological work has mapped the differences in health experience within and between populations, while setting off controversies over definition, measurement and explanation (Carr-Hill 1987). Concurrently, lay health activism stemming from contemporary social movements, such as the struggle for disability rights, the women's movement and environmentalism, has reset the agenda of work to unravel health inequalities. Increased attention has also been paid to lay knowledge and understandings of health, not as amateur or irrational by comparison with professional understandings, but as valid perspectives in their own right (Blaxter 1990; Donovan and Blake 1992). This has been reinforced by the emergence of potent qualitative research methodologies – particularly from feminist researchers (Roberts 1990; 1992). Meanwhile, there has been growing interest among medical researchers in the physiological consequences of social and environmental factors (see, for example, *British Medical Journal* 308, issue no. 6937, 30 April 1994).

This book reflects both the complexity of the evidence and the diversity of perspectives which need to be taken into account in developing understanding of the relationships between social and health inequalities. However, to date, certain broad conclusions have emerged from activity in this field.

A number of bases of disadvantage and discrimination have been revealed as being strongly associated with unequal chances and experiences of health. These are, notably, social class, relative poverty, gender, 'race', age, disability and sexual orientation (see, respectively: Townsend *et al.* 1988; Graham 1993; Ahmad 1993; Rudat 1994; Henwood 1990; Morris 1993; Quam and Whitford 1992). It is also increasingly being recognized that the experience of inequality reflects the interaction of such factors. People occupy not one but multiple social positions with consequences for health.

Meanwhile, it has become clear that these conditions which prejudice equality in health reach into all corners of people's experience of illness and health. Social inequalities affect people's life expectancy and the likelihood of their experiencing ill health (Ahmad 1993; Arber and Ginn 1993; Davey Smith *et al.* 1990; Graham 1993; King 1993; Quick and Wilkinson 1991; Townsend *et al.* 1988; Victor 1991; Woodroffe *et al.* 1993). Social inequalities affect the experience of people who are ill: the opportunities for formal diagnosis, treatment and care (Anionwu 1993; Henwood 1990); dealings with workers in formal care systems (Doyal 1994; Phoenix 1990); and the strength and availability of informal or alternative health support systems (Anderson and Bury 1988; Brotchie and Hills 1991; Patel 1993; Sharma 1992). Social inequalities affect people's opportunities to compensate for or to mask the consequences of ill health (Qureshi and Walker 1989; Williams 1993) and social inequalities also present obstacles to people trying to secure and maintain good health (Conway 1988; Blaxter 1990; Bhopal and White 1993; Graham 1993; Sooman *et al.* 1993).

A DETERIORATING SITUATION

There is, moreover, an increasing body of evidence that inequalities in Britain have been widening over at least the last decade and a half, as a result of deliberate state policy. The New Right beliefs that greater inequalities have beneficial effects in spurring on the population's economic performance, that state welfare is a damaging burden on the economy and that greater national wealth will 'trickle down' have resulted, for example, in the encouragement of wider income differentials and the tolerance of high levels of unemployment as central planks of economic planning (Milliband and Glyn 1994). Such actions as the abolition of wages councils, changes in the benefits systems affecting people who are unemployed, the sick, school leavers or pensioners and the rejection of the Social Chapter of the Maastricht Treaty on the grounds that it would place burdens on employers are all examples of this strategy (Alcock 1994; Dean 1994). Evidence of its effects have been revealed in successive analyses of the increasing divergence of income and wealth in the population (Department of Social Security 1993; Glennerster and Midgeley 1991; Joseph Rowntree Foundation 1995).

A consistent reluctance to adopt proposals to reduce other social inequalities has characterized Government action beyond the area of economic policy, for example, over immigration policy (John Baptiste 1988), racist violence (Ginsburg 1989), the age of consent for gay men (Wynn Davies *et al.* 1994), sex education in schools (Hunt 1994), community care policy (Hudson 1994; Walker and Ahmad 1994) and homelessness (Carlen 1994; Carter and Ginsburg 1994).

It is therefore not surprising that, far from improving, health inequalities in Britain appear to be increasing. There is a growing body of evidence that widening differences of income and wealth since 1980 are being reflected in widening differences in mortality between deprived and affluent groups (Davey Smith and Egger 1993; McLoone and Boddy 1994; Phillimore *et al.* 1994). Inequalities which are reflected in differential health chances are being reinforced through the changing organization of health care and treatment, for example, the privatization of health and social care (Marks 1994; Mohan 1991) and increased opportunities for profit making by the 'medical industrial complex' (Henry 1987; Stacey 1988; Worcester and Whateley 1992).

However, in the tradition of Thatcherism, current Government health strategy (Department of Health 1992) involves a deep resistance to structural understandings of, or collectivist responses to, individually experienced suffering or disadvantage (Department of Health 1989a; 1989b; Wilkinson 1991). The apparent espousal of a social model of health in *The Health of the Nation* (Department of Health 1992) proved to be an essay in placing responsibility for health maintenance and care back on the individual in the teeth of research evidence about the ineffectiveness of such an approach, derived from a programme of research commissioned and funded by the Government itself (Blaxter 1990). Unlike the World Health Organization strategy for health for all, equality was not perceived as an issue or a target (World Health Organization 1985; Davey Smith and Morris 1994).

WORK FOR GREATER EQUALITY IN HEALTH

It is against this background of powerful and interlocking tendencies that an increasing number of initiatives on the part of unpaid and paid health workers which aim to secure a more equal experience of health are being undertaken. However, as yet, little has been written which draws out the lessons from such practice. This is what this book provides. In their accounts of work in Britain and Ireland, contributors:

1 detail how their practice contributes to uncovering the processes and interrelationships through which health inequalities are maintained;
2 outline the impact of initiatives they have taken to address inequalities; and
3 draw conclusions about more effective forms of intervention.

The health workers who contribute here are drawn from a wide cross-section of occupations and write about health work undertaken in a diverse range of settings and organizations. As such they reflect the paradox that a population's health is the product of many factors, mostly outside the work of public and private health services. Indeed, most health work is the unpaid labour of lay people within their own local, primarily domestic, spheres. It is here that most preventive health work is undertaken, most illness identified, most health choices discussed and made, most treatment and care given (Graham 1984; Stacey 1988).

While perceiving the roles and insights of users and lay health workers as central to a broad strategy for tackling health inequalities, the book does not take an oppositional stance towards health and social care professionals, an increasing number of whom are equally convinced that responding to social inequalities is an essential feature of effective health care practice. Consequently the book contains accounts of the work of carers, service users and activists, whose expertise originates from personal experience of ill health and of challenging subordination and disadvantage; accounts of the efforts of health care workers to provide services which promote greater equality in health; and accounts from a variety of other contributors whose work has been centrally concerned with questions of social inequality and health.

In practice, the concerns and approaches of these three groups of workers are not discrete but resonate with each other. However, for ease of assimilation, we have chosen to group the contributions according to the common focus of their day to day work, which we have encapsulated as 'face to face care', 'redistributing resources and control' and 'information for change'.

Thus, in the early chapters contributors discuss their experience in front line health practice, whether from the perspective of a professional or a lay worker. In Chapter 2, Clare Blackburn explains how health visitors are increasingly confronting complex issues relating to poverty, such as the ways in which poverty is, for example, mediated by racism and sexism. However, legislation and policies are also reshaping health visitors' roles and responsibilities in ways that are making it difficult to respond to the health of low-income families. These changing contexts of health visiting work have challenged health visitors to develop more proactive forms of practice. Beginning with a brief analysis of the day to day experience of the recipients of health visiting services, she discusses three levels of current health visiting responses to health inequalities: monitoring; prevention and alleviation; and direct challenges to team, local and national policies that create and maintain family poverty. A consistent theme is that such responses are unlikely to bring an effective poverty perspective to health visiting unless health visitors move away from individualistic forms of practice.

In Chapter 3, Desmond O'Neill argues that attempting to tackle social inequalities should be integral to day to day 'age related health care'. The impact of social inequalities on the health of older people is evident in the populations treated by geriatricians and takes various forms. The disadvantaged position of older people is also clearly seen in the difficulties they experience after trauma such as burglary and the problems of elder abuse. Hence, O'Neill makes a case for the importance of comprehensive multidisciplinary/lay assessment, reflecting the social and psychological requirements of older people's lives and relationships, as much as issues of physical pathology or medication; for the significance for older people of access to hospital and community resources; and for geriatricians to engage in activities which raise public consciousness of ageism and specific measures required to tackle it.

Amongst social workers, too, there is a growing determination to tackle the impact of social inequalities. Paul Bywaters and Eileen McLeod, in Chapter 4, argue that social work generally, as well as explicitly health related practice (for example, hospital social work), can influence people's health, although such intervention does not necessarily result in a more equitable experience. Three examples of practice are examined, each illustrating how inequitable access to health care and resources for health can be partially redressed: first, an initiative promoting the interests of older hospital patients; second, a women's health group on an impoverished estate, which secured less stigmatizing approaches to health care; and, third, work within Social Services Departments concerned with the 'sexual health' of children in care. However, these initiatives also serve to point up the need for more fundamental shifts in resource distribution to underwrite the health and well-being of the populations concerned.

In Chapter 5, Jo Aldridge and Saul Becker shift the focus to lay health work. Drawing on qualitative research, the authors argue that the continuing invisibility of children as carers undermines the well-being of all concerned, with the effect of maintaining health inequalities.They argue that children who are undertaking primary caring responsibilities for a parent or other relatives at home, experience profound disadvantages because of their dual status as children and carers. The recipients of their 'informal' care (often their parents) also suffer by comparison with other disabled adults because they are forced to accept care – domestic, social and intimate – from their own children. Based on practical action and policy development currently being undertaken, Aldridge and Becker explore ways in which legislation and national and local professional interventions might promote the health and well-being of child carers.

The second set of chapters, which focus on redistributing resources and control, is opened by Clare Evans with a discussion of the work of the Wiltshire Community Care User Involvement Network (WCCUIN) in which she has been engaged (Chapter 6). She describes how a failure to perceive service users as co-workers can mean that health and social care professionals maintain inequalities and fail to provide services which meet users' needs. The possibility of challenging and changing this approach is demonstrated through the achievements of the Network, one of which is to have taken control over a number of services for disabled people. The range and levels of user involvement are described and an assessment made of the effectiveness of such networks in changing the attitudes of workers in health and social services towards planning and delivering services in more empowering ways.

In Chapter 7, Rosie Weaver analyses her experience as a 'locality manager' in the NHS. This provides an example of how health services management need not necessarily be geared to the promotion of internal markets in health care but can focus on the relationship between health and deprivation. Its starting point is a statistical profile of a specific locality in the Midlands, revealing the diversity of health and social needs in the area, and levels of deprivation, encompassing social divisions including ethnicity, gender and age. A range of initiatives taken within the locality to confront the social inequalities revealed in this profile are then discussed. Lessons and directions for future work at a local level and an assessment of what it is possible to achieve locally, emerge from these initiatives.

In Chapter 8, Simon Sedgwick-Jell explores the role local councils can play by developing policies and services which contribute to equalizing health chances. Through a discussion of three diverse projects concerning house insulation and heating, the effects of transport policy on pollution and the impact of compulsory competitive tendering on workers' health, he demonstrates the possibility of local government recapturing its historical role in the field of public health, if necessary in opposition to central government policy.

The preceding chapters raise questions about the extent to which there may be common or linked health interests between paid health workers (and their managers) and users of health services. On these grounds the significance of public service trades union strategies for securing a more equitable experience of health is analysed. In Chapter 9, Mick Carpenter reviews the organization of community care, and the role of trades unions within it, in the context of the transformation of community care since 1945 and specifically of the New Right-inspired restructuring of the local state. He examines two main ways in which unions have responded to the populist promotion of consumer involvement, first by demystifying the rhetoric of the reforms, showing that they will result in widespread rationing and privatization, and, second, by campaigning for alternative services through which employed workers and users and carers can be jointly empowered.

The unions' role in providing alternative sources of information about what is happening to health services is one issue discussed by Carpenter. In the final section, the place of research and the dissemination of information in combating health inequalities is examined further. Nick Spencer, in Chapter 10, discusses some of the key lessons which have emerged from recent epidemiological studies for his practice as a paediatrician and the importance of paediatricians becoming directly involved in research aimed at changing social and health policy as it impacts on the health chances of children and young people.

In Chapter 11, Hilary Graham illustrates how sociological research can also contribute to the development of new policies for tackling health inequalities. The example she explores is that of research into an aspect of lay health care: the lives of women on income support caring for children. In the long-running policy debates about inequalities in health, individual behaviour and social conditions have been represented as two mutually-exclusive categories of explanation. Yet, as she shows, everyday accounts of health and illness point to the inter-connections between lifestyles and living conditions and suggest that the routines through which mothers work to promote health are developed in resistance to the material circumstances in which they are caring for their children.

Graham's chapter concludes by arguing that this research evidence goes against the continuing emphasis of health promotion policies on giving more information and more advice. Instead, it makes the case for welfare policies and services which act directly on the social and material conditions in which mothers in low-income households are working to keep their children healthy and their families together. In Chapter 12, Jenny Douglas describes such an approach to health promotion, exploring the role it can play in opposing the impact of racism and racial discrimination on the health of Black people in the United Kingdom. She discusses ways in which health can be maintained in Black communities, against a backcloth of social determinants resulting from racism, such as poor housing, poverty, unemployment and poor working conditions. After presenting information about the differential health experience and health status of Black communities, the chapter analyses examples of local health promotion projects. These examples expose the links between poverty, racism and health, highlight gaps in service provision for Black communities and demonstrate the need to encourage the participation of voluntary organizations and community groups in determining appropriate methods for health promotion.

Finally, in Chapter 13, Simon Watney examines the significance of work done, primarily within the gay community, to wrest control from researchers and health professionals over the production and dissemination of knowledge about HIV and AIDS. He draws on his involvement in the emergence of newsletters in the US and Europe aimed at providing lay access to reliable, up-to-date information about clinical trials and other aspects of potentially useful treatment drugs, as a strategic response to the absence of a proper national government plan for the management of the epidemic, and as a means for drawing people into 'treatment activism' more generally. The chapter concludes by raising the question of whether such work in the AIDS/HIV field provides a model for the relationships of other 'disease communities' with the medical and pharmaceutical industries.

LESSONS FROM PRACTICE

Several key findings emerge from these accounts. First, the accounts corroborate existing understandings of the experience of health inequalities in three ways.

1 The contributions repeatedly underline the difficulties many people face in securing the basic material resources which would provide the necessary foundation for reasonable health – shelter, warmth, food, social interaction and personal care. It is not the objective of this book to make the case for linking relative poverty with poor physical health, psychological malaise, disability or premature death – that has already been established. (See, for example, Blaxter 1990; Smith and Jacobsen 1988; Quick and Wilkinson 1991.) But, in describing their work, contributors consistently reflect in detail the impact of poverty on people's health; including the ways in which low income is commonly linked to other deficits in resources such as the absence of good quality housing, leisure facilities, health and social services and reduced opportunities for education and employment.

2 The study provides further evidence of the interwoven nature of different strands of inequality and discrimination. The contributors do not simply reflect the fact that poverty is more widespread amongst particular groups of the population, they document the existence of additional barriers to health equality, for example, institutionalized racism, sexism and ageism. They recount how attitudes to disabled people, gays or lesbians, single parents, people with learning disabilities or those in the care system may also lead either to stigma and victim blaming or to invisibility and marginalization. Moreover, they record the kaleidoscopic way in which a range of dimensions to inequality undermines the health of individuals and populations.

3 The accounts illustrate the interactive nature of psychological and physical well-being. There has been growing evidence that a lack of the material resources necessary to promote or maintain health negatively affects emotional as well as physical health and, clearly, poor physical and emotional health can feed one another (Blaxter 1990; Graham 1993; McLeod 1994; Wilkinson 1994). In these chapters, contributors describe the experience of working with, or being part of, populations who battle on to obtain physical well-being, but who tend to do so in isolation, such as children caring for disabled parents, women parenting on income support and frail older people living alone. Unsupported, members of these populations are at risk of anxiety, fatalism and dejection. The contributors document how those concerned face not only the rigours of emotional suffering but increased risks of physical ill health arising from their lowered emotional state.

Second, the book is a testimony to the powerful negative impact on health of two of the main planks of current Government policy.

1 For the most part, the accounts focus on action by individuals and groups of workers within local geographical communities or communities of interest. Again and again the well-being of such communities was being further jeopardized by the withdrawal of material resources consequent on central government measures. Moreover, reduced funding for public services in real terms curbed initiatives to equalize health chances: schemes to create healthier living and working environments or to develop access to health care services were thwarted; more realistic provisions for personal care with benefits for whole families were at best subject to short-term and shoestring funding. In summary, this study demonstrates

that central government commitment to equalizing the quality and level of material resources is integral to the health interests of populations and the population at large.

2 The authors reveal the deep significance for initiatives addressing health inequalities of the effects of changes in the ideology and in the organization and management of welfare provision. The consequences of the shift towards market-based, targeted and means-tested public services, towards intensifying managerial and budgetary controls over professional activity and towards privatized, 'domesticated' and commercialized alternative services is clearly visible in the extent to which diverse populations experienced increasing difficulties in obtaining the prerequisites of health and in the extent to which the initiatives described here are localized, provisional, at risk of being disregarded and vulnerable to being swept away.

Against these odds, in a dominant climate of oppressive material and ideological conditions – which may persist irrespective of changes of administration – activity within local communities and communities of interest to secure greater equality in health may seem doomed to failure and therefore to irrelevance. However, the studies provide a variety of forms of evidence that focused or local initiatives can achieve health gains for populations; both through the immediate help they bring and through developing 'pockets of resistance' to prevailing inegalitarian ideas and circumstances. Moreover, analyses presented here of the outcomes of attempts to map and dissolve health inequalities suggest that certain initiatives do offer a chance of greater purchase on the problem.

Third, the book sets out proposals for action to secure greater equality in health. Common themes in these proposals are:

1 Lay health work, rather than the work of professionals on their own, is central to the development of challenges to dominant ideas, relations, institutions and practices, which undermine an equitable experience of health. Whether through asserting rights and needs, through providing mutual support and encouragement, through struggles for better working conditions, through gaining control over information about health, through educating professionals, through obtaining changes in service provision or by securing improved material circumstances, the achievements of lay activism are writ large in these chapters.

2 In turn this raises questions about the nature of the relationship

between lay health workers and health professionals and other paid health workers. Conventional health and social care practice was frequently experienced by the recipient population as dominating, exploitative or amounting to forms of rationing or policing, in short, as not acting in the interests of their health. Thus in some accounts professionals and paid staff were the targets for change, although in others, it was paid health workers who instigated action on behalf of and/or with the population concerned. The presence or emergence of hierarchies within lay activity was also apparent.

The contributors suggest the potential benefits of alliances between lay, professional and other paid health workers based on a common commitment to eradicating health inequalities and on a developing and shared analysis. However, in doing so the contributors also highlight that the complexity of the social relations involved requires engagement with a set of taxing issues. First, acknowledgement of difference between the respective parties which may reflect differing material and social positions. Second, the development of adequate support for and recognition of health work whatever its current status and location. Third, the gradual discovery of sets of health interests which are genuinely held in common, viz., freedom from air pollution. Finally, the dissolution of crude notions of separate roles within health work. In any one day an individual may move between being an unpaid carer, paid health worker, lay health worker and service user.

3 The book also illustrates how practice aiming to secure a more egalitarian experience of health can and should make common cause with action on disability rights. As things stand, these two spheres of activity and analysis tend to be set apart. However, our study makes it clear that strategically the two issues are indissoluble. The contributors highlight, for example, the intimate connection between the requirements of disabled people and the needs of informal and paid carers and demonstrate how failure to meet these requirements prejudices the health and well-being of all three parties. Moreover, they demonstrate how similar forms of action need to be undertaken to reverse the processes whereby social inequality is manifest in ill health and disability. These include: developing greater understanding of the nature and social origins of the suffering involved, building co-operative working alliances across lay and professional lines, acquiring the resources to underwrite such initiatives and beginning to bring about significant shifts in resources and power relations in the interests of disadvantaged groups.

4 The studies demonstrate that it is crucial to take account of the interactive nature of psychological and physical well-being in trying to dissolve health inequalities. The encouragement and development of self-confidence and self-esteem through advocacy, self-help or collective action was pivotal to people becoming more assertive in pursuing their requirements for physical and psychological well-being, in negotiation with more powerful interests. This applied whether in the case of paid workers encouraging older patients to apply for services, of disabled users *vis à vis* a social services department or of gay activists *vis à vis* the medical research establishment. Making such a point is not to disregard the psychological demands which ill health or the fear of ill health intrinsically generates. It is to demonstrate the crucial part played by collective activism in fostering psychological well-being in order to relieve unnecessary suffering.

5 Finally, our contributors demonstrate that, in three respects, action for a more equitable experience of health is indissolubly linked with wider social/economic action to secure more equitable social relations *per se*. First, health initiatives discussed here repeatedly emanate from the influence of wider social movements such as civil rights for Black and disabled people, the contemporary women's movement and gay and lesbian activism. Moreover, a central objective of such activism has been to obtain resources for care, health maintenance and recovery, such as services, job opportunities and benefits, as a right, rather than, at best, on a discretionary basis. Second, the fate of the initiatives discussed here demonstrates their inextricable links with central government's commitment and ability to secure decent levels, and the equitable distribution nationally, of material resources in the context of movements of international capital. Third, the evidence across the chapters here is that incremental gains in securing a more equitable experience of health arising from focused or local initiatives may feed into the creation of demands for, and a constituency with a vested interest in, more equitable social relations generally.

CONCLUSION

Throughout these proposals for more effective action to address health inequalities, it is not assumed that health problems would vanish with the establishment of substantially greater equality nor that only such a goal is worth pursuing. While the creation of just social relations and an equal distribution of goods might arguably be the biggest single contribution which could be made to the health of the population, it would not end the personal and social impact of disease and death. Nevertheless, the health workers' accounts presented here indicate that tackling the impact of social inequalities on health is a necessary part of the prevention and relief of unnecessary suffering, which is the crux of health work.

Paradoxically, the accounts also reveal that, to be effective, action for health has to incorporate or accommodate more centrally, skills and forms of practice not conventionally considered a part of health work. Prominent among these are:

1 surveying the incidence and nature of factors associated with health inequalities and disability across populations and unravelling the causal connections;
2 elaborating economic strategies on a local and nationwide basis, to equalize material well-being;
3 developing greater understanding of the interactive nature of social inequalities and the effects of these on health and disability and undertaking initiatives which begin to resolve them; and
4 developing co-operative, collective working alliances across lay/professional divides in pursuit of more equitable living conditions.

Finally, as the work of all the contributors demonstrates, social inequalities are not just powerful, external influences on people's lives. Through our experience of health and illness, inequalities are lived out physically and psychologically: they take bodily form in our everyday lives. Our bodies are a site of oppressive social relations. Through this volume we hope to make a small contribution to understanding how health inequalities occur, are maintained but may be combated.

REFERENCES

Ahmad, W.I.U. (ed.) (1993) *'Race' and Health in Contemporary Britain*, Milton Keynes: Open University Press.
Alcock, P. (1994) 'The end of the line for social security: the Thatcherite restructuring of welfare', *Critical Social Policy* 40: 88–105.
Anderson, R. and Bury, M. (eds) (1988) *Living with Chronic Illness*, London: Unwin Hyman.
Anionwu, E. (1993) 'Sickle cell and thalassaemia: community experiences and official response', in Ahmad, W.I.U. (ed.) *'Race' and Health in Contemporary Britain*, Milton Keynes: Open University Press.

Arber, S. and Ginn, J. (1993) 'Gender and inequalities in health in later life', *Social Science and Medicine* 36 (1): 33–46.

Bhopal, R. and White, M. (1993) 'Health promotion for ethnic minorities: past, present and future', in Ahmad, W.I.U. (ed.) *'Race' and Health in Contemporary Britain*, Milton Keynes: Open University Press.

Blaxter, M. (1990) *Health and Lifestyles*, London: Routledge.

Brotchie, J. and Hills, D. (1991) *Equal Shares in Caring*, London: Socialist Health Association.

Carlen, P. (1994) 'The governance of homelessness: legality, lore and lexicon in the agency-maintenance of youth homelessness', *Critical Social Policy* 41: 18–35.

Carr-Hill, R. (1987) 'The inequalities in health debate. A critical review of the issues', *Journal of Social Policy* 16: 509–42.

Carter, M. and Ginsburg, N. (1994) 'New government housing policies', *Critical Social Policy* 41: 100–8.

Conway, J. (ed.) (1988) *Prescription for Poor Health*, London: London Food Commission, Maternity Alliance, SHAC, Shelter.

Davey Smith, G. and Egger, M. (1993) 'Socioeconomic differentials in wealth and health: widening inequalities in health', *British Medical Journal* 307: 1085–6.

Davey Smith, G. and Morris, J. (1994) 'Increasing inequalities in the health of the nation', *British Medical Journal* 309: 1453–4.

Davey Smith, G., Bartley, M. and Blane, D. (1990) 'The Black Report on Socioeconomic Inequalities in Health Ten Years On', *British Medical Journal* 301: 373–7.

Dean, H. (1994) 'Recreating the void: the November 1993 Budget', *Critical Social Policy* 41: 109–16.

Department of Health (1989a) *Working for Patients*, London: HMSO.

—— (1989b) *Caring for People: Community Care in the Next Decade and Beyond*, London: HMSO.

—— (1992) *The Health of the Nation: A Strategy for Health in England*, London: HMSO.

Department of Social Security (1993) *Households Below Average Income: A Statistical Analysis 1979–1990/1*, London: Government Statistical Service.

Donovan, J.L. and Blake, D.R. (1992) 'Patient non-compliance: deviance or reasoned decision-making', *Social Science & Medicine* 34 (5): 507–13.

Doyal, L. (1994) 'Changing Medicine? Gender and politics of health care', in Gabe, J., Kelleher, D. and Williams, G. *Challenging Medicine*, London: Routledge.

Ginsburg, N. (1989) 'Racial harassment policy and practice: the denial of citizenship', *Critical Social Policy* 26: 66–81.

Glennerster, H. and Midgeley, J. (eds) (1991) *The Radical Right and the Welfare State: An International Reassessment*, London: Harvester Wheatsheaf/Barnes and Noble Books.

Goodman, A. and Webb, S. (1994) *For Richer For Poorer: The Changing Distribution of Income in the United Kingdom, 1961–91*, London: Institute For Fiscal Studies.

Graham, H. (1984) *Women, Health and the Family*, London: Harvester Wheatsheaf.
—— (1993) *Health and Hardship in Women's Lives*, London: Harvester Wheatsheaf.
Henry, F.J. (1987) 'Violence against women: the pharmaceutical industry', *Free Enquiry in Creative Sociology* 15 (2): 199–205.
Henwood, M. (1990) 'No sense of urgency – age discrimination in health care', in McEwan, E. (ed.) *Age – The Unrecognised Discrimination*, London: Age Concern.
Hudson, B. (1994) 'Independent living for people in Britain with a severe disability: too successful by half? The case of the Independent Living Fund', *Critical Social Policy* 40: 88–96.
Hunt, L. (1994) 'Sex education curbs will mean more pregnancies', *Independent*, 30 March: 2.
John Baptiste, M. (1988) 'The implications of the new Immigration Bill', *Critical Social Policy* 23: 62–9.
Joseph Rowntree Foundation (1995) *Enquiry into Income and Wealth*, York: Joseph Rowntree Foundation.
King, E. (1993) *Safety in Numbers*, London: Cassell.
McLeod, E. (1994) 'Patients in inter-professional practice', in Soothill, K., Mackay, L. and Webb, C. (eds) *Interprofessional Issues in Health Care*, London: Edward Arnold.
McLoone, P. and Boddy, F.A. (1994) 'Deprivation and mortality in Scotland, 1981 and 1991', *British Medical Journal* 309: 1465–70.
Marks, L. (1994) *Seamless Care or Patchwork Quilt? Discharging Patients from Acute Hospital Care*, London: King's Fund Institute.
Milliband, D. and Glyn, A. (eds) (1994) *Paying For Inequality: The Economic Costs of Social Injustice*, London: Rivers Oram Press.
Mohan, J. (1991) 'Privatization in the British health sector: a challenge to the NHS?', in Gabe, J., Calnan, M. and Bury, M. (eds) *The Sociology of the Health Service*, London: Routledge.
Morris, J. (1993) *Independent Lives? Community Care and Independent Living*, Basingstoke: Macmillan.
Patel, N. (1993) 'Healthy margins: Black elders' care – models, policies and prospects', in Ahmad, W.I.U. (ed.) *'Race' and Health in Contemporary Britain*, Milton Keynes: Open University Press.
Phillimore, P., Beattie, A. and Townsend, P. (1994) 'Widening inequality of health in northern England, 1981–91', *British Medical Journal* 308: 1125–32.
Phoenix, A. (1990) 'Black women and the maternity services', in Garcia, J., Kilpatrick, R. and Richards, M. (eds) *The Politics of Maternity Care*, Oxford: Clarendon Press.
Quam, J.K. and Whitford, G.S. (1992) 'Adaptation and age-related expectations of older gay and lesbian adults', *The Gerontologist* 32 (3): 404–13.
Quick, A. and Wilkinson, R. (1991) *Income and Health*, London: Socialist Health Association.
Qureshi, H. and Walker, A. (1989) *The Caring Relationship*, Basingstoke: Macmillan.

Roberts, H. (ed.) (1990) *Women's Health Counts*, London: Routledge.
—— (1992) *Women's Health Matters,* London: Routledge.
Rudat, K. (1994) 'Black and minority ethnic groups in England, health and lifestyles', London: Health Education Authority.
Sharma, U. (1992) *Complementary Medicine Today*, London: Routledge.
Smith, A. and Jacobson, B. (1988) *The Nation's Health: A Strategy For the 1990s*, London: King Edward's Hospital Fund.
Sooman, A., Macintyre, S., and Anderson, A. (1993) 'Scotland's health – a more difficult challenge for some? The price and availability of healthy foods in socially contrasting localities in the West of Scotland', *Health Bulletin* 51: 276–84.
Stacey, M. (1988) *The Sociology of Health and Healing*, London: Unwin Hyman.
Townsend, P., Davidson, N. and Whitehead, M. (1988) *Inequalities in Health: The Black Report and the Health Divide*, London: Harmondsworth, Penguin.
Victor, C. R. (1991) *Health and Health Care in Later Life*, Milton Keynes: Open University Press.
Walker, R. and Ahmad, W. (1994) 'Window of opportunity in rotting frames? Care providers' perspectives on community care and black communities', *Critical Social Policy* 40: 46–9.
Wilkinson, R.G. (1991) 'Inequality is bad for your health', *Guardian*, 12 June.
—— (1994) 'Divided we fall', *British Medical Journal* 308: 1113–14.
Williams, S.J. (1993) *Chronic Respiratory Illness*, London: Routledge.
Woodroffe, C., Glickman, M., Barker, M. and Power, C. (1993) *Children, Teenagers and Health: The Key Data*, Buckingham: Open University Press.
Worcester, N. and Whateley, M.J. (1992) 'The selling of HRT: playing on the fear factor', *Feminist Review* 41, Summer: 1–26.
World Health Organization (1985) *Targets for Health for All: Targets in Support of the European Regional Strategy for Health for All*, Copenhagen: World Health Organization Regional Office for Europe.
Wynn Davies, P., Brown, C. and Macdonald, M. (1994) 'Sexual equality for gays rejected', *Independent*, 2 February: 1.

Chapter 2

Building a poverty perspective into health visiting practice

Clare Blackburn

For health visitors, providing services to people in poverty is nothing new. Indeed, like other community workers, their origins lie in a concern to improve the health of low-income families (Lewis 1980). While providing community health services amid increasing poverty and health inequalities continues to be a core feature of health visiting work, health visitors are also aware that legislation and policies are reshaping their roles and responsibilities in ways that make it increasingly difficult to respond to the health needs of low-income clients. This changing context of health visiting work has challenged some health visitors to develop more proactive forms of practice.

This chapter seeks to explore some of the ways in which health visitors have attempted to move away from individualistic forms of practice towards responses that locate people's health experiences and the effects of poverty on it within a structural analysis. It will begin with a brief discussion of family poverty levels in the United Kingdom, concentrating on the position of families with young children as the main user group of health visiting services. It will then move on to discuss some current health visiting responses that seek to combat health inequalities. It will address three broad types of responses: profiling and monitoring; preventing and alleviating; working for social change. A theme of this discussion is that building a more overt poverty perspective into all health visiting work is central to developing effective health visiting responses to tackle social inequalities in health. This, in turn, is dependent on moving away from individualistic forms of practice, towards team work approaches.

THE BACKDROP TO HEALTH VISITING WORK

The pressures on health visitors to respond more effectively to poverty and its associated health costs have been sharpened since the early 1980s by changes to the material position of families with young children. A feature of the 1980s and early 1990s has been the increasing burden of poverty placed on the shoulders of families with dependent children. The *Household Below Average Income* statistics indicate that poverty levels have increased sharply among this group (Department of Social Security 1993). Between 1979 and 1991, the number of households with dependent children with incomes of less than 50 per cent of average income rose from 3.4 million (12 per cent of the population) to 7 million (28 per cent of the population). High levels of unemployment and low pay appear to have hit families with dependent children particularly hard so that they now form the largest single group in poverty. In 1991, families with children made up more than half of the poorest 10 per cent of the population, compared to a third three decades ago (Goodman and Webb 1994).

Poverty, however, is unequally distributed between different groups and individuals within groups. Lone-parent families, particularly those headed by women, appear especially vulnerable to poverty. Two-thirds of the income of lone-parent households comes from benefits (Goodman and Webb 1994). Black families, as a group, not only have a higher proportion of dependent children than the population as a whole, itself associated with poverty, but they also have poorer access to the labour market, particularly to well-paid and secure jobs (Amin and Oppenheim 1992). Families including disabled people also appear to experience higher poverty levels than other families. The Office of Population Censuses and Surveys (OPCS) 'Disability Survey' found that a third of families with a disabled adult had incomes less than half the average income compared to a quarter of families without disabled adults (Martin and White 1988).

An increase in the number of families in poverty has been accompanied by a deterioration in the financial circumstances of individual families. Goodman and Webb's analysis of the changing distribution of income in the UK suggests that the real incomes of the poorest tenth of the population, after housing costs, fell sharply between 1961 and 1991, representing a return to the living standards of a quarter of a century ago (Goodman and Webb 1994). Over the last decade, studies have been documenting, on the one hand, the difficulties associated with caring for family health in poverty (see, for example, Graham in this volume), and, on the other hand, how low income and poverty shape the health and health experiences of adults and children (Quick and Wilkinson 1991; Wilkinson 1994). Income appears to be a key health resource for families, shaping their access to other important health resources, including healthy housing, safe environments, healthy food and supportive networks of family and friends.

The scale of poverty in the United Kingdom means that promoting health in poverty is a core feature of health visiting work. While not all health visitors work in areas of high deprivation and disadvantage, the majority of health visitors have at least some low-income families on their caseloads. In some areas, however, some health visitors may have caseloads where 90 per cent of the families they work with are in receipt of means-tested benefits. A considerable amount of health visiting time and resources then, are spent working with families experiencing the social and material hardships and the health costs of poverty. As poverty and its health costs appear to be inextricably bound to health visiting work, it would seem crucial that health visiting services are constructed in ways that have a positive impact on the lives of low-income users.

Health visiting has its historical roots in the nineteenth-century visiting movements concerned with reducing infant mortality rates among working-class families (Prockoska 1980). The literature which describes the activities of the early health visitors suggests that their work was concerned with poverty (for example, see Abbot and Sapsford 1990). A review of the health visiting literature relating to a period from the 1950s to the early 1980s indicates far less concern with the social and material conditions associated with health (for example, see McEwan 1962; Owen 1977). This period appears to represent a shift towards developing universal service provision for families regardless of income or social and material conditions and a growing concern with the individual health behaviour and the responsibilities mothers have for family health. The professional literature and documents relating to the profession during this time make few references to poverty and health inequalities.

Following the publication of the Black Report (Townsend and Davidson 1982) and the introduction of a new literature and set of debates on social inequalities in health in the late 1970s and 1980s (for example, see Townsend 1979; Graham 1984; Whitehead 1987), a concern with poverty and deprivation appears to have crept back into health visiting and is visible within health visiting texts, journals and reports (for example, see Luker and Orr 1985; Goodwin 1988;

Twinn and Cowley 1992; Blackburn 1992a). This renewed interest in poverty and health inequality issues is reflected in the work of a growing number of practitioners who, since the mid-1980s, have been developing new ways of working with families and communities in poverty in recognition that traditional forms of response, based on changing the behaviour of individuals, are likely to have little impact on the health or well-being of families in poverty.

Across the UK, health visitors are responding in a variety of ways to the challenge of family poverty and health inequalities. This range of responses reflects, on the one hand, the diversity of poverty experiences across social groups and localities and, on the other hand, the complexity of the day to day working environments of health visiting teams across localities, Health Authorities and Community Trusts.

Blackburn (1992b) has identified three broad types of health visiting responses that are central to positive support strategies for families in poverty: profiling and monitoring responses that seem to gather and analyse information on family poverty as aids to planning and working for social change; preventing and alleviating responses that seem to help families to avoid, mitigate and cope with the material and health effects of poverty; and social change responses that seem to directly challenge team, local and national policies that create and maintain family poverty. Using this broad typology here, it is possible to illustrate some of the key ways in which some health visitors are responding to the challenge of tackling poverty and health inequalities in their daily practice.

PROFILING AND MONITORING THE EFFECTS OF POVERTY

Profiling and monitoring the impact of poverty on the health of families and communities appears to be a key part of any proactive health visiting responses. Without information on local poverty levels and the health and social costs of poverty for individuals and families, health visiting teams are unlikely to be able to evaluate the effectiveness of current strategies or make judgements about how they should be responding to poverty and health issues. Nor will they be able to monitor changes in family circumstances in a locality or how these changes affect families' health and well-being.

While profiling the health of local communities has been an integral part of health visiting for some years, it has often been an isolated activity, seen as an end in itself rather than as one linked to other areas of practice. More recently, it is evident that health profiling has been given renewed emphasis and is beginning to be used as a basis for developing more responsive health visiting strategies. This process has been driven partly by a recognition within health visiting of a need to move away from universal provision towards a locality-, needs-based approach and by the realization that poverty and health profiles have the potential to drive the health care purchasing process.

While many profiles document the extent of health problems and health inequalities in localities and comment on the social and material circumstances within which people live, they often fail to incorporate a specific poverty perspective. However, the recognition that poverty and health issues have been actively screened out of debates about health inequalities and commissioning has led to attempts by some health visiting teams to establish an explicit poverty perspective in their work. Several models of health profiling are evident within health visiting. While those that predominate tend to be based on workload and caseload profiling, other models are emerging that move towards more community approaches to health needs assessment.

One such model has been developed by the Strelley health visiting team in Nottingham. Recognizing the value of a public health approach, the Strelley team have evolved a model whereby one member of the team has taken on a specific remit for co-ordinating health profiling activities under a broader umbrella of public health work. Profiling activities have been given greater legitimacy through the creation of a specific post within the team and have been based on the deliberate building in of a poverty focus. The profile collects and co-ordinates information on the local population's health status by focusing on the level of poverty and its impact on family health and well-being (Boyd et al. 1993). Profiling activities are seen as on-going and the profile is regularly updated to take account of new changes and new information. While one team member co-ordinates the collection of information, other team members are actively involved in developing the profile and in analysing the information. The team feel that as well as exposing the level and extent of poverty in the area, the profile has given them a greater insight into unmet health and social need within the locality, exposing unmet needs such as poor nursery provision for the under fives, lack of safe play areas and inadequate welfare rights services. Importantly, the health profile has been seen as an essential tool for planning, developing and evaluating services and work strategies have evolved from health profile information.

The Strelley team have recognized that involving local people in the profiling process is central to developing a poverty perspective to their work. In the process of revising the health profile, local groups are being consulted about their health needs and views about services. A health profiling model based on work with local people to identify health need in an area of high unemployment has been described by O'Gorman and Moore (1990). The Blackstaff community health profile in Belfast was co-ordinated by a local health visitor with a community worker and research worker, but involved a wide range of community groups. Local groups participated in the identification of topics to include in the profile and have been involved in collecting profile information.

The health profiling work described here raised some important issues relating to the current roles and responsibilities of health visitors, suggesting that some investment in building local networks and alliances with local groups and individuals is of great value and central to health profiling work. Building alliances and networks requires time, and needs to be recognized and made legitimate by purchasers through service contacts. Similarly, health authorities need to ensure the continuation of poverty and health profiling through the contacting process. While some health authorities recognize the value of this, others have yet to support this work.

PROVIDING PREVENTIVE AND ALLEVIATING SERVICES

For many low-income families, there is little hope that their circumstances will change for the better in the near future. Providing services that assist families to avoid, mitigate and cope with the material and health effects of breadline living seems important. It's easy to dismiss ameliorative responses as trivial, but for many families they are crucial. Providing empowering, sensitive and supportive responses rather than victim-blaming at a time of continuing social and economic difficulties for families is valuable in itself and can be combined with more proactive strategies that work for social change.

Central to alleviating/preventing responses is assisting families to maximize their access to material and social resources for health. Billingham's study (1993) of health visitors' interactions with low-income mothers suggests that many health visitors do actively work to increase women's resources directly and through advocacy work. Assisting families to maximize their incomes through helping them to claim benefits they are eligible for would appear to be an important aspect of health visiting. Some evidence suggests that in addressing financial difficulties, health visitors may attempt to do so in terms of money management rather than in terms of the money available to families (Edwards and Popay 1994). Given that research suggests that the majority of families manage their money well (Kempson *et al.* 1994) it would seem that working to maximize incomes rather than money management is the issue for health visitors to address. In some Community Trusts, asking about benefits status and assessing to see if families need to be referred on for welfare rights advice is standard practice for health visitors. In others, however, questions about income and benefits are left to the discretion of individual workers, who may screen out poverty issues in their contacts with clients through failure to raise the issue, often on the basis that asking questions about sources of income is intrusive.

Maximizing access to other social and material resources is also a feature of the work of some health visitors. Innovative work has been carried out by the Stepney Neighbourhood Nursing Team. As part of their public health project, the team have been actively trying to improve people's access to local resources for health. Based on a 'rights model' rather than traditional health promotion models, the team are working on housing issues (James and Buxton 1994). They have negotiated training in housing issues which has led to a number of outcomes. With the collaboration of housing lawyers, rights workers and a local General Practitioner practice, a weekly housing clinic has been established at a health centre offering advice, guidance and advocacy to local people. The team have also made a joint bid with Neighbourhood Energy Action for funding to support a project on fuel poverty. This multi-agency project aims to provide bilingual training for workers in the locality involved in community work to help local people to improve fuel efficiency and obtain resources to improve insulation.

While poor take-up of services by low-income families itself is not a cause of health inequalities, it is likely to contribute to the maintenance of health inequalities. If health visitors are to assist families to avoid and cope with some of the most serious health effects of poverty, then services need to be offered at easily accessible venues and in a format that is culturally and socially acceptable to families. Several examples of increasing service accessibility and acceptability can be seen in the work of the Stepney Neighbourhood Nursing Team. Having developed a link with an Asian Women's Group, they provide a weekly health visitor/ linkworker drop-in clinic for local Bangladeshi women. Uptake of developmental assessments for children has increased to 100 per cent since this service was offered and the location of the clinic within the women's group has had other broader outcomes, including the development of a nutrition project to work on a more participatory approach to supporting healthy weaning grounded in the beliefs and perspectives of the local community (James and Buxton 1994).

Making services more accessible and acceptable is also a theme of workers at the Cope Street Project in Nottingham. Since 1987, the health visitors together with midwives and nursery workers have been providing group support and health care in a rented house for young mothers living in an inner-city area (Rowe 1993). Main users of the project's facilities are lone mothers on Income Support, parenting in difficult housing circumstances. An evaluation of Cope Street's work indicates that the project is successful in making services more accessible and acceptable to a group of women who often fail to use traditional services (MacKeith et al. 1991).

WORKING FOR SOCIAL CHANGE

While preventing and alleviating responses appear to be crucial to families in poverty, they need to be coupled with responses that seek to challenge team, local and national policies that create and maintain family poverty. Examples of good practice of this type of response are much harder to find, but they do exist. For example, the Stepney team have combined preventing and alleviating responses with more active social change work on housing issues, campaigning to raise awareness of the links between poor housing and health among local people and politicians (James and Buxton 1994).

Effective social change responses appear to develop out of profiling and monitoring activities. For example, in response to information on home accidents and a lack of safe play areas, the Strelley health visiting team have worked for the development of a home safety equipment scheme for low income parents and have facilitated community involvement in the planning and trial of traffic calming measures in the locality (Boyd et al. 1993). Health visiting support for a parents' campaign for safe play facilities has also been described by Blackburn (1991) and is not atypical of work in this area.

Profile information has also been used by health visitors to secure other social and material resources for local people. The Strelley team community health profile also highlighted the need for appropriate and accessible welfare rights advice. Using profile information, the team were able to gain the support of local councillors to secure the funding of additional welfare rights services in the locality (Strelley Nursing Development Unit 1994).

Transferring skills and information to local people so that they can work to secure resources for their communities appears to be another important area of work that can develop out of profiling and monitoring activities. The Blackstaff community health profile described earlier in this chapter led to a number of initiatives within the community, including the setting up of a community transport co-operative and successful community action on smoke hazards in the local area (O'Gorman and Moore 1990).

Other examples include the Stepney Neighbourhood Nursing Team's Children's Public Health/Mental Health Project. Through work with local children, this project aims to demonstrate children's rights to influence local public health policy and decisions about the provision of community child health services. Based on a child empowerment model, it will use audio-visual materials to document the environmental and public health issues linked to children's mental health (James 1994).

PROACTIVE HEALTH VISITING RESPONSES: SOME KEY FEATURES

In drawing out the core features of the proactive and innovative responses described above, it is possible to identify a team approach and management support as key aspects of health visiting responses that attempt to tackle health inequalities. Traditionally, health visitors have worked, on the whole, as individual workers with individual families, deciding on their own priorities within the broad strategy of the organization in which they work. While the *Health of the Nation* strategy (Department of Health 1992), local health targets and the priorities of General Practitioner fundholders have all limited health visitors' perceived freedom to work on their own priorities, many health visitors continue an individualistic mode of practice.

The work of the health visitors described in this chapter highlights the centrality of a teamwork approach to practice in the area of poverty and health inequalities. Team work appears to allow health visitors to build more integrated and flexible local responses out of an examination of team attitudes, knowledge and local circumstances. Good teamwork is most likely to develop out of team building. Working in teams does not necessarily come naturally and can be suffused with tensions (Boyd and Brummell 1993). It has been demonstrated that using a team training approach can enable teams of health visitors to incorporate a specific poverty perspective into their work and lead to more effective team work (Blackburn 1993).

The examples discussed here suggest that where teams have been able to develop, team working allows the members' range of skills and resources to be channelled to benefit local people. In the words of the Strelley health visitors, it enables teams to 'develop shared objectives with a shared vision' (Strelley Nursing Development Unit 1994). As well as facilitating more effective work within the team, such an approach may also lead to more effective work with other workers. In several of the examples discussed here, health visitors have recognized from an analysis of the locality health profiles that developing joint responses with other agencies in the area is important when working on structural issues like poverty.

Teams have also documented how a teamwork approach can improve morale within the team and produce a more stable unit (Strelley Nursing Development Unit 1994). Working on health inequality issues is fraught with difficulties and tensions which may result in inaction and a perceived sense of helplessness (Blackburn 1993). Areas of high material and social deprivation frequently have a high turnover of health visitors and difficulty recruiting staff. This, coupled with the presence of workers on short-term funded projects, often results in little continuity of care for local people or cohesive and co-ordinated work on a long-term basis. Clearly, strategies that stabilize the workforce are more likely to contribute to the long-term health gain of families than those that destabilize.

Management support also seems to be a key factor in the development of responsive services for people in poverty. The majority of the projects described here have active management support at both Community Trust and locality level. Innovative work is only likely to be successful and integrated into mainstream work if managers are willing to allow practitioners to move away from traditional forms of practice to test out new ideas and ways of working. Managers in provider units act as intermediaries between purchasers and front-line practitioners and, unless they are willing to provide purchasers with information about the value and benefits – in both the long and the short term – to the local population, these innovative responses are unlikely to secure resources, either by direct funding or within the broader service contracts.

As the main organizational unit for primary health care becomes the primary health care teams linked to General Practitioner (GP) practices, it may well become more difficult for health visiting and community nursing teams to develop or maintain the type of locality-based responses described here. This is particularly likely to be the case as more GPs become fundholders and thus purchasers of health visiting services, able to dictate service contract specifications. For many health visitors and their managers, the challenge is how they can balance the individualized child and family health issues, frequently the main concern of many GPs, with the more collective public health work described in this chapter.

The response of the Strelley and the Stepney teams to this challenge has been to develop a community-based approach with links to primary health care teams. But both of these teams have the advantage of being designated Nursing Development Units, receiving grants to support innovative work. In both cases this has facilitated the developments of the public health side of their work. These additional funds have been used to provide extra clinical leadership, evaluation activities and bank cover to allow team members to participate in training and planning activities. Essentially, it provides them with the thinking and planning time not usually available. But as test-beds for new ideas, they do enable pilot work to be carried out before changes are introduced into other teams. Clearly, a commitment within purchasers' contracts to allow health visiting and primary health care teams thinking and planning time is crucial.

CONCLUSION

The scale of poverty in the UK means that a large proportion of health visiting time is spent working with families with children in poverty. Building a poverty perspective into all aspects of health visiting work is the key to developing more effective health visiting strategies. This, in turn, appears to be dependent on moving away from traditional, individualized ways of working and towards team work approaches. The evidence discussed in this chapter suggests that when health visitors provide services that are flexible and responsive to the needs of families with dependent children they can help families avoid some of the worst aspects of poverty and health inequalities. At best, they may even be able to provide a challenge to policy makers to develop strategies that reduce poverty and health inequalities.

Within the limits of this chapter, it is only possible to offer a flavour of some of the ways in which health visitors across the UK are responding to health inequalities and family poverty. While some types of work such as working to maximize resources for families appear to be fairly common across health visiting, other responses appear to be isolated examples of good practice. Many of the more proactive and innovative responses to poverty and health issues described here are short-term funded projects lying outside mainstream health visiting. The task facing health visitors is to seek ways of anchoring this type of work within mainstream health visiting work, with mainstream funding.

REFERENCES

Abbot, P. and Sapsford, R. (1990) 'Health visiting: policing the family?', in Abbot, P. and Wallace, C. (eds) *The Sociology of the Caring Professions*, London: Falmer Press.

Amin, K. and Oppenheim, C. (1992) *Poverty is Black and White: Deprivation and Ethnic Minorities*, London: Child Poverty Action Group.

Billingham, K. (1993) 'Love costs nothing: a study of health visitors' interactions with mothers living in poverty', unpublished MA thesis, Coventry: University of Warwick.

Blackburn, C. (1991) 'The Boxhill parents' group', in Child Accident Prevention Trust *Preventing Accidents to Children: A Training Resource for Health Visitors*, London: Health Education Authority.

—— (1992a) *Poverty Profiling: A Guide for Community Nurses*, London: Health Visitors' Association.

—— (1992b) 'Family poverty: what can health visitors do?', *Health Visitor* 64 (11): 368–70.

—— (1993) 'Making poverty a practice issue', *Health and Social Care* 1 (6): 297–305.

Boyd, M. and Brummell, K. (1993) 'Working as a team', *Primary Health Care* 3–5, Grasping the Nettle Supplement: 3–4.

Boyd, M., Brummell, K., Billingham, K. and Perkins, E. (1993) *The Public Health Post at Strelley: An Interim Report*, Nottingham: Strelley Nursing Development Unit.

Department of Health (1992) *The Health of the Nation: A Strategy for Health in England*, London: HMSO.

Department of Social Security (1993) *Households Below Average Income:*

A Statistical Analysis 1979–1990/1, London: Government Statistical Service.

Edwards, J. and Popay, J. (1994) 'Contradictions of support and self-help: views from providers of community health and social services to families with young children', *Health and Social Care* 2 (1): 31–40.

Goodman, A. and Webb, S. (1994) *For Richer For Poorer: The Changing Distribution of Income in the United Kingdom, 1961–91*, London: Institute for Fiscal Studies.

Goodwin, S. (1988) *Whither Health Visiting?*, London: Health Visitors' Association.

Graham, H. (1984) *Women, Health and the Family*, Brighton: Wheatsheaf Books Ltd.

James, J. (1994) Personal Communication, December 1994.

James, J. and Buxton, V. (1994) *Stepney Nursing Development Unit Annual Report 1994*, London: Stepney Nursing Development Unit.

Lewis, J. (1980) *The Politics of Motherhood: Child and Maternal Welfare in England 1900–1939*, London: Croom Helm.

Luker, K. and Orr, J. (1985) *Health Visiting*, London: Blackwell Scientific Publications.

Kempson, E., Bryson, A. and Rowlingson, K. (1994) *Hard Times? How Poor Families Make Ends Meet*, London: Policy Studies Institute.

MacKeith, P., Phillipson, R. and Rowe, A. (1991) *45 Cope Street, Young Mothers Learning through Group Work: An Evaluation Report*, Nottingham: Nottingham Community Health.

McEwan, M. (1962) *Health Visiting: A Textbook for Health Visitor Students*, London: Faber and Faber.

Martin, J. and White, A. (1988) *The Financial Circumstances of Disabled Adults Living in Private Households in Britain, OPCS Survey of Disability in Britain, Report No.2*, London: HMSO.

O'Gorman, F. and Moore, S. (1990) 'Two tales of a healthy city', *Health Visitor* 63 (8): 276–8.

Owen, G. (1977) *Health Visiting*, London: Bailliere Tindall.

Prockoska, F. (1980) *Women and Philanthropy in Nineteenth-Century England*, Oxford: Clarendon.

Quick, A. and Wilkinson, R. (1991) *Income and Health*, London: Socialist Health Association.

Rowe, A. (1993) 'Cope Street Revisited', *Health Visitor* 66 (10): 358–9.

Strelley Nursing Development Unit (1994) *Changing Needs: Changing Minds, Changing Practice*, Nottingham: Strelley Nursing Development Unit.

Townsend, P. (1979) *Poverty in Britain*, Harmondsworth: Penguin.

Townsend, P. and Davidson, N. (1982) *Inequalities in Health: The Black Report*, Hardmondsworth: Penguin.

Twinn, S. and Cowley, S. (1992) *The Principles of Health Visiting: A Re-examination*, London: Health Visitors' Association.

Whitehead, M. (1987) *The Health Divide: Inequalities in Health in the 1980s*, London: Health Education Council.

Wilkinson, R. (1994) *Unfair Shares: The Effects of Widening Income Differences on the Welfare of the Young*, Ilford: Barnardos.

Chapter 3

Health care for older people

Ageism and equality

Desmond O'Neill

INTRODUCTION

Although those who live by the crystal ball may be condemned to die by eating broken glass, one sure forecast is the increase not only in the number and proportion of those aged over 65, but particularly those over the age of 80, in both developing and developed nations. This is a result of the alteration of two prime characteristics of undeveloped societies, high rates of fertility and mortality. Contrary to widespread public opinion, this change has very little to do with high-tech medicine keeping older people alive for ever longer periods. As the main determinants have been social improvements and preventive medicine, the absolute and relative numbers of older people are rising in the developing world. The increase seen in developed nations will be mirrored in developing nations: older people's homes have appeared already in several capital cities in South East Asia (Phoon *et al.* 1983). The World Health Organization has forecast that there will be 600 million people over the age of 60 in the world by the year 2000: two-thirds of these will be in the developing world, as opposed to 50 per cent in 1960 (World Health Organization 1989).

Despite this increase in the worldwide population of older people, there is evidence that ageist attitudes and ageist social conditions, in interaction with other dimensions to social inequality such as poverty and sexism, continue to undermine older people's health. This chapter highlights this phenomenon. It then discusses, with reference to Britain and Ireland, how medical care can reinforce such an inequitable situation, before examining in general and specific terms how geriatricians can contribute to eradicating ageism and thereby help to secure a better experience of health for older people.

OLDER PEOPLE'S SURVIVAL – AGEIST ATTITUDES AND UNEQUAL LIVING CONDITIONS

A major debate has focused on whether this greatly increased number of older people will result in an overwhelming burden on the health and social services. For example, while older people constitute 12 per cent of the population of the United States, older patients consume 33 per cent of total health expenditure (US Senate Special Commission on Ageing 1988). However, many who speak in gloomy terms of 'demographic time bombs' or 'greying of the nations' lack perspective on the major advances of another revolution earlier this century, that of the reduction of child mortality. One in two Victorian children died in the first eight years of life: this fact was accepted by society as normal. Pioneering paediatricians faced a battle reminiscent to that of early geriatricians to prioritize the fight against childhood diseases. They did not concentrate only on the medical problems of childhood but they also acted as powerful advocates for change in social attitudes and conditions which were responsible for so much ill health and misery in the earlier part of this century. In developed countries, childhood is no longer an obstacle course in which half of the children fall at the hurdles. This major success story should provide an encouraging example for those contemplating the demographic changes of the late twentieth century.

A further alarmist view point, depicting ageing as a threat, queries the ability of future generations to support an increasingly numerous elderly population financially. This anxiety has been fuelled by an inappropriate reliance on population dependency ratios. These may be divided into those aged over 65 (gerontic dependants) and those aged 0–15 years (neontic dependants) as a ratio of those aged 16–64 years. Several contentious and ageist assumptions are made, particularly that all those aged 16–64 are gainfully employed while all those aged 0–15 and over 65 are 'dependent'. Older people may point out that they are not just passive recipients and play an important role in reducing the cost of ageing. Over 40 per cent of carers providing more than 50 hours of support a week to an older person are themselves retired (Victor 1991). It is also worth noting that the numbers over age 65 increased by one third between 1961 and 1981 in the United Kingdom without causing an intergenerational war for resources.

The question of access to income in later life is also complex, reflecting the heterogeneity of old age. It relates to such factors as country, age, gender and pre-retirement socio-economic status.

While people aged 65–74 in the United States and several northern European states enjoy incomes which represent 94 per cent of that of the population average, the corresponding figure for the United Kingdom is 76 per cent (Hedstrom and Ringen 1987). On the one hand, there is growing evidence that a certain proportion of older people seem to have benefited reasonably well from changes in benefits and pensions that have occurred. The argument has developed to the point that there is now a movement in the United States complaining that older people consume a disproportionate share of the collective income by way of health and social benefits (Johnson 1992)! This argument may reflect more on the poor levels of such care afforded to younger, economically disadvantaged people, particularly in the United States, rather than on a supposedly ample level of care for older people (Wisendale 1988).

The opposing position is that any changes reflect an extremely low base line to start with: for example, people at retirement age in the UK represented 50 per cent of those in the lowest income group in 1971, despite being less than 15 per cent of the population. In 1984 they represented 16 per cent of the population and still were over-represented in the lowest income group, but this proportion had fallen to 22 per cent (Jefferys 1992). There are also considerable income differentials between older people. Some evidence suggests that the extremes of social isolation and poverty amongst older people represent a cohort effect and that these trends may be less pronounced in future generations of older people (Victor 1991). However, there is evidence of growing income inequalities amongst the older population across the past decade, mirroring that of the population at large. The incomes of the richest fifth of pensioners grew by 40 per cent during the 1980s: those of the poorest fifth rose by only 5 per cent (Hancock and Weir 1994). Many frail older people are in the most impoverished group of society and completely dependent on state benefits. Those at most risk of significant poverty include those over the age of 80, women, those living alone and disabled elders (Victor 1991). Such poverty constrains day to day choices which are central to health maintenance. For example, a survey for Age Concern has found that increases in the Value Added Tax on fuel have led to 37 per cent of pensioners at the lowest income level reducing the amount they spend on food and clothing in order to find the extra money to pay fuel bills (Age Concern 1995).

Discrimination and disadvantage also persists into later life in other ways which prejudice health. For example, discrimination on grounds of ethnicity presents obstacles to access to resources for social care (Markides *et al.* 1990; Ahmad 1993). There is also only a minimal literature on gay and lesbian sexual orientation among older people, and my own experience is that the issue of sexual orientation may be ignored despite social and clinical relevance (O'Neill *et al.* 1988; O'Neill 1992a).

THREATS TO OLDER PEOPLE'S WELL-BEING FROM WITHIN HEALTH SERVICES

Despite some improvements in the lives of older people, as outlined above, many are disadvantaged. Various processes within health care delivery tend to further disadvantage older people. Levels of physical impairment are at their highest among older people (Hunt 1978). This is nearly always a sign of a disease which, acute or chronic, may respond to medical intervention and the input of social or material resources. However, the narrow focus of an over-specialized medical model of health is such as to place a low priority on the assessment (not to mention remediation) of physical impairment among older patients. Studies of the detection of physical impairment among older patients in general medical and surgical wards have shown very low pick-up rates: for example, that only 9 per cent of the incidence of physical impairment was noticed by doctors, and 27 per cent by nurses (Ryall *et al.* 1994). Undetected physical or psychological impairment cannot be responded to.

Discrimination against older people or ageism in the provision of health care services (Currie 1987), in the form of a 'triple whammy', also undermines health. First, discrimination in the health services includes restricted access to services such as coronary care units (despite evidence that this resource is more effective in older people than in younger people) (Dudley and Burns 1992), cancer therapy (Fentiman *et al.* 1990) and kidney transplantation in the United Kingdom. Second, negative and discriminatory attitudes are very widely held within the health care professions and are easily passed on to students (O'Neill *et al.* 1990). Third, many patients and their carers suffer from unconscious ageism, suffering stoically from conditions while ascribing them to 'old age'. If a 40-year-old woman could not get out of her chair unaided, it is unlikely that she or her family would accept a diagnosis of 'middle ageing' and accept the provision of a hoist, meals-on-wheels and a home help! Just as paediatrics has reversed a fatalism towards child mortality, so geriatricians must try to combat a nihilistic approach to physical impairment in later life, among the general population.

THE AGE RELATED HEALTH CARE TEAM – A MEANS OF COMBATING DISADVANTAGE?

Currently one of the key features of geriatric medicine is the emphasis on team work. Increasingly this is described as inter-disciplinary rather than multidisciplinary. One of the major texts on establishing a geriatric medical service (Coakley 1981) lays major emphasis not only on team work but also on the liaison between the service and the community and, in particular, social and community services. There has also been a trend to alter the name of the service to reflect the team approach, away from 'geriatric medicine' to alternative titles, often chosen to avoid the pejorative connotations of 'geriatric': indeed 'elderly' or 'old' may be little better. Our own department name, Age Related Health Care, was decided after a survey of patients, marketing managers and journalists (O'Neill *et al.* 1993). For convenience, geriatric medicine and dedicated ser-vices for the provision of health care of older people will from now on be referred to as age related health care (ARHC).

The development of a cohesive and effective interdisciplinary style is one of the major challenges facing ARHC. The inter-disciplinary team required is often large, including the patient, family/carers, nurses, doctors, physiotherapists, occupational therap-ists, social workers and dieticians as a core group. This group will often call upon the services of psychologists, chiropodists, pastoral care, psychiatrists, other medical and surgical specialities and also liaise with the community services. There is a strong emphasis on multi-faceted assessment and remediation and growing evidence as to its effectiveness as an approach to health in later life (Rubenstein and Rubenstein 1992). As Dr Johnson might have remarked, the wonder is not that it is done well, but that it is done at all.

There is a developing literature on the workings of the inter-disciplinary team, but empirical data is scarce. Our own experience is that a problem with detection of physical or psychological impairment persists (albeit at a lower level than on general wards) despite weekly interdisciplinary case conferences and journal clubs (Cunningham *et al.* forthcoming). Our proposed solution is to try to develop regular audit, review and continuing team education in issues related not only to each discipline's expertise in contributing to health in later life but also to referral patterns among ourselves. An interesting design problem for us was to consider what measures we would use to assess team members' knowledge of the need for social work intervention. Situations where social work intervention is required cannot be compressed into standard formulae. Moreover, there is considerable variation in how social workers define their role: just as doctors may range from monospecialists to holistic practitioners, an outsider might perceive a range of styles within social work, from almoner to committed political activist. The position of the social worker in the interdisciplinary team has been discussed by McLeod (1994): among the useful initiatives outlined is greater encouragement of self-referral to social work by patients.

An even less clearly developed part of team practice is the participation of the patient and family/carers. Apart from the obvious fact that they are the clients/service users, the success or failure of rehabilitation depends very much on the participation of patient and carers as well as the goals being acceptable to them. For example, it has been shown that interpersonal obstacles are the main determinant of loss of independence three years after a stroke: i.e., it is not the physical impairment which is crucial, but the extent to which the patient leaves tasks to the carer, or to which the carer takes over tasks unnecessarily from the patient (Söderback and Caneman 1993). The patient and carer are also the only team members without formal training, and this may leave them feeling vulnerable and powerless. Fortunately, it is increasingly recognized in clinical practice that lack of progress in rehabilitation stems from a range of causes which include dissonance between the goals of patients and professionals, undiagnosed depression, dementia and perceptual impairment and from a range of social factors, such as fear of returning home.

POSITIVE CHARACTERISTICS OF ARHC

At its most positive, the following measures characterize the work of the ARHC team with older people.

1 Providing access for the patient to a range of services that work in a reasonably co-ordinated fashion to provide assessment, treatment, rehabilitation and return to the community where practicable. This service understands that assessment, treatment and management is a multi-layered process. It is necessary to treat not only the damaged system in the body (for example, the injury

to the brain in stroke) but also the rest of the body (which may be at risk), to take account of psychological attitudes of patients and carers and to institute changes in the physical environment (ranging from adaptations making clothing easier to put on right through to access to the shops) to the patient's advantage (Tallis 1992). Rehabilitation also involves mobilizing a social support network, including both formal carers and statutory agencies, in the patient's favour.

2 Providing an advocacy service for individual patients (especially those compromised by impairment, both physical and cognitive) and for groups of patients. For example, access to coronary care units has been fought largely by geriatricians rather than cardiologists. Much ageism stems from ignorance about the value of these interventions in later life. ARHC services have been at the forefront in demonstrating that many of these interventions are not only extremely cost-effective in later life but also that it is not that much more difficult to apply them. Another key example is the cost effectiveness of total hip replacement in later life (Wilcock 1981). Similarly, in the first few hours after a heart attack, many older people have previously been excluded from therapy which dissolves the clot in the artery (Hendra and Marshall 1992). A major international study showed that in fact older people gain more benefit from this therapy than younger people. However, it was common practice up until the early 1990s not to administer clot-dissolving therapy to older people following heart attacks. It took the pioneering work of geriatricians like Hendra to demonstrate that it was practical, feasible and effective to tackle the problems associated with giving this medication and that it is possible to ensure a higher uptake. Access to coronary care units ironically is still limited in some centres in the UK and geriatricians have been keen to publicize this through academic publications (Dudley and Burns 1992).

3 Training students in all health care professions to view health care provision for older people in a positive and constructive way. There is evidence to suggest that this approach can modulate negative perceptions and encourage positive attitudes towards older people (Peach and Pathy 1982). It is encouraging that many general practitioner training schemes rotate trainees through ARHC units.

4 Collaborating with, supporting and providing appropriate training for patients and their carers. In our own unit this takes place at three levels. On an individual basis, carers are invited to join in

the rehabilitation process at an early stage so that they are aware of the processes involved and can participate. At a second level, various members of the interdisciplinary team participate in an eight-week carer training programme run by the Eastern Health Board in Dublin. This involves a series of informal talks, with plenty of time for question and answer sessions. Finally, we are running an experimental training programme for the carers of patients with dementia, in six afternoon sessions.

5 Contributing to greater recognition of the need to alleviate the problem of women, mainly, being caught up in balancing the requirements for personal care of children and parents as well as themselves. This is now recognized as an issue in the ARHC literature (Shapiro 1991). Geriatricians have also been instrumental in the development of innovative schemes to support older people and their carers. For example, being induced to recognize that the stress of caring for an older relative can affect an employee's work performance (Creedon 1991), has led several North American corporations to institute elder care programmes to support carers. These include measures ranging from telephone helplines to day care facilities (*Fortune Magazine* and John Hancock Financial Services 1989). Carer support groups also represent an important initiative by carers to ensure their needs feature in measures for the care of older people. Integration of these groups into ARHC teams requires greater flexibility on the part of ARHC teams as well as training programmes for both carers and the teams.

6 Combating alarmist views, often expressed by such phrases as 'the demographic time bomb', which portray older people as relentless consumers of scarce resources.

7 Highlighting to policy makers issues of social, medical and political significance which have an impact on the quality of life of older people: for example, the elder abuse position paper from the British Geriatrics Society (British Geriatrics Society 1992).

8 Researching the complex phenomena of the interactions between ageing, disease and social circumstances in such issues as burglary and fitness to drive (as will be discussed later).

ARHC – SPECIFIC EXAMPLES OF INITIATIVES COMBATING DISADVANTAGE

The development of health care which takes account of the complex interaction between health, social circumstances and wider community issues in addressing specific aspects of older people's health is critical if ARHC is actually to contribute to a postive experience of health for older people. Two specific examples of this are now discussed: the devastating effect of burglary on older people (O'Neill 1990) and a positive view of fitness to drive (O'Neill 1992b).

The impact of burglary on older people

This issue illustrates the role that ARHC teams have in bringing key health issues to public attention.

The first case report on crime and older people in the medical literature was published in 1979 (Coakley and Woodford-Williams 1979). This demonstrated how simple burglary can have a devastating impact and outlined how violation of the privacy of the home seems to have a particularly unsettling effect on older people's perception of the home as a secure base. It also described how patients reported a degree of morbidity that greatly exceeded that which might be expected from previously existing physical illness. Although comparative crime studies have shown that older people in general are not particularly at risk of burglary (Van Dijk et al. 1991), at least two subsequent studies have indicated that non-violent crime such as burglary has a particularly harmful effect on older people (Chew and Cheshire 1989; O'Neill et al. 1989). They have shown that older people in such situations are considerably more prone than younger controls to suffer from a wide range of medical, social and psychological after-effects. These include hospitalization, institutionalization, a reduction in mobility, sleep disorders, anxiety, depression and fear of going out (O'Neill et al. 1989). These features may be familiar to any health worker who is involved with the care of older people in the community.

Once the serious problem of the impact of burglary on older people's physical and psychological well-being is recognized, predisposing factors for victimization can be established and used to develop preventive measures, as well as strategies to address the consequences. There is mounting evidence that increasing rates of crime are closely associated with increasing poverty and unemployment (Wells 1995). While long-term solutions to the problem of burglary confronting older people may therefore be out of ARHC teams' hands, encouraging short-term preventive measures and publicizing the relatively acute consequences for older people appropriately lie within ARHC teams' remit. Amongst older people several risk factors have been identified as being associated with victimization. These include frailty, social isolation (alone by day and by night), impaired mobility, an overtrusting attitude to callers and lack of security equipment (O'Neill *et al.* 1989). In those cases where frailty or vulnerability is irreversible, certain initiatives can compensate for these factors. There is some evidence to suggest that older people living in sheltered housing may be less vulnerable to burglary (Chew and Cheshire 1989), and this form of housing should be encouraged. Alarm and alert systems have been relatively under-used, although pilot schemes have shown them to be effective in promoting emergency contact with the relevant services (Department of Health 1986). The over-trusting attitude of many older people to callers could be countered both by encouraging vigilance among older people and by ensuring that representatives of public services present proof of identity routinely when visiting. Doctors and paramedical staff should also provide identification at the first home visit and the practice of leaving doors open for community health workers should be discouraged.

Provision of security aids in the houses of older people seems to be very inadequate in published surveys: in one study of older people in Birmingham, over 40 per cent had no mortice lock on their front door (Centre for Applied Gerontology 1988). State or local govern-ment financial help may be necessary as the provision of even simple security aids may be beyond the purse of many pensioners. Despite increasing emphasis on purpose-built housing for older people, planning of such housing may not allocate sufficient priority to simple security measures: provision of such measures is important if older people are to remain in the community. A comprehensive and useful set of guidelines has been published for builders, housing authorities and older people themselves (Centre for Applied Geron-tology 1989). However, all these factors should be approached as part of a more comprehensive plan as emphasis on security alone could encourage a siege mentality (Clemente and Kleiman 1979).

Potential offenders should also be targeted: male adolescents feature prominently in convictions for burglary (House of Commons Home Affairs Committee 1993). Education programmes in schools outlining the potentially disastrous consequences of burglary on older people may deter some crime against this age group.

Responses to older people who are burgled also need to incorpor-ate education of the police in the serious implications of even minor crime for older people. The police are very often the first point of contact for older people after a burglary, and concern and re-assurance are important even when the incident is very 'minor' or when hope of resolution of the case is minimal. Early contact with medical and community services is also indicated. Meanwhile medical and paramedical personnel need to be educated to take the problem seriously and to intervene rapidly in such cases (O'Neill 1990). The use of victim support groups may prove to be a very useful aid to normalization among older victims as well and guidelines for the formation and running of such groups are available (Age Concern Action against Crime Advisory Group 1980).

In summary, burglary against older people has been recognized only recently as an important hazard for older people living in the community, which may severely compromise their ability to live independently. As with other such hazards, for example, hypo-thermia, recognition of the seriousness of the phenomenon is the first step towards dealing with the problem adequately and ARHC teams have a key role to play in this.

Fitness to drive

Car ownership and use is related to income and gender (Graham 1993). Nevertheless, there is evidence that older people who own cars are also being restricted from using what is generally recognized as a key social asset, on ageist and disablist grounds.

Maintaining social contacts, getting to appointments, access to health care and shopping are among the primary functions of driving in older age groups: 77 per cent of drivers over the age of 55 perceive driving as essential or very important (AA Foundation for Road Safety Research 1988). Loneliness among older people is correlated with the loss of driving ability (Berg et al. 1981). Notwithstanding issues of environmental pollution, it has been agreed that continued driving in later life should be welcomed as sign of integration into society (Eisenhandler 1990).

However, not only are doctors generally unaware of the regu-lations of fitness to drive for many illnesses in later life (O'Neill et al. 1994), but these regulations are couched in language that is predominantly negative (Medical Advisory Branch 1994). There is only a minuscule literature on enabling older people to drive. This is despite evidence that many of those who suffer from a stroke, for example, not only stop driving, but are not offered either driving assessment or remediation (Legh-Smith et al. 1986). The evidence for restricted driving in many illnesses is at best controversial and a proactive approach to driver training may further increase driver safety and reduce insurance premiums (Malfetti and Winter 1986). It is important that more training should be given to general practitioners and hospital doctors about the importance of driving to older people and that older patients should be routinely questioned about driving practices, as much as about continence or mobility. Any training schedule during undergraduate and postgraduate medical training concerning fitness to drive should accentuate the positive aspects of the physician's role and base any decisions for restricted driving on solid evidence. A typical illness with potential for enabling is arthritis. Patients experience many difficulties in driving (Thevenon *et al*. 1989), but there is also evidence to show that appropriate intervention may improve driving ability and comfort (Jones *et al*. 1991).

A scheme of assessment which has proved useful in practice is to divide the driving task into three components: strategic, tactical and operational (O'Neill 1993). Strategic performance includes the planning of choice of route, time of day (avoiding rush hour), or even the decision not to drive and to take public transport. Tactical decisions are those aspects of the driving style which are characteristic of the driver and are consciously or unconsciously adopted for a great range of reasons, for example, decisions on whether or not to overtake or go through amber lights or signalling in good time before turning. Operational performance is the response to specific traffic situations, such as speed control, braking and signalling. Driving a car requires organization of action at all three levels.

Assessment up to now has tended to dwell on deficiencies on the operational level, i.e., whether an illness affects the subject's appreciation of distracting stimuli or the reaction time to a hazardous situation. This emphasis is misguided: reaction time (a measure which is an integral part of operational tasks) is shortest in the 15–25 year age group, the group with the highest accident rate. It is very likely that decisions at a strategic and a tactical level are much more important in causing accidents. Older drivers are known to use strategic and tactical measures widely, for example, to avoid delay, stress and risk by driving less at night and during bad weather, avoiding rush hours and unfamiliar routes (AA Foundation for Road Safety Research 1988; Michon 1989). Wider dissemination of this approach may spare some older people from the catastrophe of not being able to drive.

CONCLUSION

While ageing at the end of the twentieth century is characterized by a relative improvement in the health and income of many older people, a significant proportion are not only affected by multiple illnesses and are disabled but also find themselves extremely dependent financially and discriminated against – including by traditional medical structures. The challenge of ARHC teams is to move beyond working as an assessment and rehabilitation team in the classical sense. Instead there is the need to involve the patient and carer as co-workers; to develop an interdisciplinary approach embodying the development of a shared language of care; and to adopt an evangelical approach against ageism and other elements of disadvantage faced by older people. As the foregoing discussion has shown, it is also important for ARHC teams to forge working relationships with organizations and institutions not customarily considered as partners in health care. These include the involvement of town planners and transportation consultants in providing positive environments to encourage independent living, and lobbying against ageism in society in conjunction with voluntary bodies such as Age Concern. In these ways ARHC teams may contribute to realizing the full extent of late life potential.

REFERENCES

AA Foundation for Road Safety Research (1988) *Motoring and the Older Driver*, Basingstoke: AA Foundation for Road Safety Research.
Age Concern (1995) News Release 8.2.95: 'Gallup Poll Shows Poorer Pensioners Cut Back on Basics To Pay Fuel Bills', London: Age Concern.
Age Concern Action against Crime Advisory Group (1980) *Victim Support Schemes*, Mitcham, Surrey: Age Concern.
Ahmad, W.I.U. (ed.) (1993) *'Race' and Health in Contemporary Britain*, Buckingham: Open University Press.
Berg, S., Mellstron, D. and Persson, G. (1981) 'Loneliness in the Swedish aged', *Journal of Gerontology* 36: 342–9.
British Geriatrics Society (1992) *Elder Abuse*, London: British Geriatrics Society.
Centre for Applied Gerontology (1988) *Security in the Homes of the Elderly, Report of a Survey*, Birmingham: Centre for Applied Gerontology.
——— (1989) *Report of the Working Party on Security in the Homes of Elderly People*, Birmingham: Centre for Applied Gerontology.
Chew, C. and Cheshire, C.M. (1989) 'Effects of burglary on elderly people', *British Medical Journal* 299: 516.
Clemente, R. and Kleiman, M.B. (1979) 'Fear of crime among the aged', *Gerontologist* 16: 211–19.

Coakley, D. (ed.) (1981) *Establishing a Geriatric Medical Service*, London: Croom Helm.

Coakley, D. and Woodford-Williams, E. (1979) 'Effects of burglary and vandalism on the health of old people', *The Lancet* ii: 1066–7.

Creedon, M. (1991) 'Economic consequences of Alzheimer's disease', in O'Neill, D. (ed.) *Carers, Professionals and Alzheimer's Disease*, London: John Libbey.

Cunningham, C., Hogan, F., Connolly, P., Mannion, A. and O'Neill, D. (forthcoming) 'Detection of disability by different members of a multidisciplinary team in a geriatric rehabilitation setting', *Irish Journal of Medical Science*.

Currie, C.T. (1987) 'Doctors and ageism', *British Medical Journal* 295: 1586.

Department of Health (1986) *Communication Networks and the Elderly*, Dublin: Department of Health.

Dudley, N.J. and Burns E. (1992) 'The influence of age on policies for admission and thrombolysis in coronary care units in the United Kingdom', *Age and Ageing* 21: 95–8.

Eisenhandler, S.A. (1990) 'The asphalt identikit, old age and the driver's licence', *International Journal of Ageing and Human Development* 30: 1–14.

Fentiman, I.S., Tirelli, U., Monfardini, S., Schneider, M., Festen, J., Cognetti, F. and Aapro, M.S. (1990) 'Cancer in the elderly, why so badly treated?', *The Lancet* 335: 1020–2.

Fortune Magazine and John Hancock Financial Services (1989) *Corporate and Employee Response to Caring for the Elderly, a National Survey of US Companies and the Workforce*, New York: The Time Magazine Company & John Hancock Financial Services.

Graham, H. (1993) *Hardship and Health in Women's Lives*, London: Harvester Wheatsheaf.

Hancock, R. and Weir, P. (1994) *More Ways than Means, a Guide to Pensioners' Incomes in Great Britain during the 1980s*, London: Age Concern.

Hedstrom, P. and Ringen, S. (1987) 'Age and income in contemporary society, a research note', *Journal of Social Policy* 16: 227–39.

Hendra, T.J. and Marshall, A.J. (1992) 'Increased prescription of thrombolytic treatment to elderly patients with suspected acute myocardial infarction associated with audit', *British Medical Journal* 304: 423–5.

House of Commons Home Affairs Committee (1993) *Juvenile Offenders, Vol. 1*, London: HMSO.

Hunt, A. (1978) *The Elderly at Home*, London: HMSO.

Jefferys, M. (1992) 'The elderly in society', in Brocklehurst, J.C., Tallis, R.C. and Fillit, H.M. (eds) *Textbook of Geriatric Medicine and Gerontology*, Edinburgh: Churchill Livingstone.

Johnson, M. (1992) 'Intergenerational equity', *Review of Clinical Gerontology* 2: 79–81

Jones, J.G., McCann, J. and Lassere, M.N. (1991) 'Driving and arthritis', *British Journal of Rheumatology* 30: 361–4.

Legh-Smith, J., Wade, D. and Hewer, R.L. (1986) 'Driving after a stroke', *Journal of the Royal Society of Medicine* 79: 200–3.

McLeod, E. (1994) 'Patients in interprofessional practice', in Soothill K., MacKay, L. and Webb C. (eds) *Interprofessional Relations in Health Care*, London: Edward Arnold.

Malfetti, J.L. and Winter, D.J. (1986) *Drivers 55 Plus, Testing your Own Performance*, Washington: AAA Foundation for Road Safety.

Markides, K.S., Liang, J. and Jackson, J.S. (1990) 'Race, ethnicity and ageing, conceptual and methodological issues', in Markides, K.S., Liang, J. and Jackson, J.S. (eds) *Handbook of Ageing and the Social Sciences*, San Diego: Academic Press.

Medical Advisory Branch D. (1994) *At a glance leaflets*, Swansea: DVLA.

Michon, J.A. (1989) 'Explanatory pitfalls and rule-based driver models', *Accident Analysis and Prevention* 21: 341–53.

O'Neill, D. (1990) 'Crime and the elderly', *Journal of the Irish Colleges of Physicians and Surgeons* 19: 18–19.

—— (1992a) 'HIV and the elderly', *Journal of the Royal Society of Medicine* 85: 712.

—— (1992b) 'Physicians, elderly drivers and dementia', *The Lancet* 339: 41–3.

—— (1993) 'Illness and elderly drivers', *Journal of the Irish College of Physicians and Surgeons* 22: 14–16.

O'Neill, D., Crosby, T., Haigh, R., Shaw, A. and Hendra, T. (1994) 'Physician awareness of driving regulations for older drivers', *The Lancet* 344: 1366–7.

O'Neill, D., Daly, S., O'Carroll, S., Rice, I., Walsh, J.B. and Coakley, D. (1990) 'Attitudes to geriatric medicine among students and doctors', *Irish Journal of Medical Science* 159: 118.

O'Neill, D., O'Neill, J., Walsh, J.B. and Coakley, D. (1988) 'HIV seropositivity in a geriatric medical unit', *Postgraduate Medical Journal* 64: 832.

O'Neill, D., Rice, I., Walsh, J.B. and Coakley, D. (1993) 'What's in a name?' *Journal of the American Geriatrics Society* 41 (Suppl): SA67.

O'Neill, D., O'Shea, B., Lawlor, R., McGee, C., Walsh, J.B. and Coakley, D. (1989) 'Effects of burglary on elderly people', *British Medical Journal* 298: 1618–19.

Peach, H. and Pathy, M.S. (1982) 'Attitudes towards the care of the aged and to a career with elderly patients among students attached to a geriatric and general medical firm', *Age and Ageing* 11: 196–202.

Phoon, W.O., Tan, S.B. and Tye, C.Y. (1983) 'A study of the residents of five old people's homes in Singapore', *Community Medicine* 5: 38–49.

Rubenstein, L.A. and Rubenstein L. (1992) 'Multidimensional geriatric assessment', in Brocklehurst, J.C., Tallis, R.C. and Fillit, H.M. (eds) *Textbook of Geriatric Medicine and Gerontology*, Edinburgh: Churchill Livingstone.

Ryall, N., Connolly, P., Namushi, R. and O'Neill, D. (1994) 'Detection of functional disability in older patients in the acute hospital', *Irish Journal of Medical Science* 163 (Supplement): 21.

Shapiro, B.A. (1991) *The Big Squeeze, Balancing the Needs of Ageing Parents, Dependent Children and You*, Bedford, MA: Mills & Sanderson.

Söderback, I. and Caneman, G. (1993) 'Causes of dependence in personal care after stroke', *NeuroRehabilitation* 3: 60–71.

Tallis, R.C. (ed.) (1992) *The Clinical Neurology of Old Age*, Wiley: Bristol.

Thevenon, A., Grimbert, P., Dudenko, P., Heuline, A. and Delcambre, B. (1989) 'Polyarthrite rhumatoïde et conduite automobile', *Revue de Rhumatisme* 56: 101–3.

US Senate Special Commission on Aging (1988) *Aging America, Trends and Projections, 1987–88 edition*, Washington, DC: United States Department of Health and Human Resources.

Van Dijk, J., Mayhew, P. and Killias, M. (1991) *Experiences of Crime Across the World*, Amsterdam: Kluwer.

Victor, C. (1991) *Health and Health Care in Later Life*, Milton Keynes: Open University Press.

Wells, J. (1995) *Crime and Unemployment*, London: Employment Policy Institute.

Wilcock, G.K. (1981) 'A comparison of total hip replacements in patients aged 69 years or less and 70 years or over', *Gerontology* 27: 85–91.

Wisendale, S.K. (1988) 'Generational equity and intergenerational policies', *Gerontology* 28: 773–8.

World Health Organization (1989) 'Health of the elderly, report of a WHO expert committee', *World Health Organization Technical Report Series* 779: 14–31.

Chapter 4

Can social work deliver on health?
Paul Bywaters and Eileen McLeod

SOCIAL WORK, HEALTH AND INEQUALITY

Social workers in the United Kingdom work primarily with people who are living in poverty, compounded by disadvantage on the grounds of disability, age, gender, sexual orientation and ethnic identity. These conditions – heavily implicated in a higher incidence of physical and psychological ill health (see Chapter 1) – are reflected in the high levels of physical and psychological morbidity amongst users of social work services (Clare and Corney 1982; Cumella 1994; Shaw 1991).

Hitherto, evidence of social work's impact on the health of service users has come mainly from the analysis of practice in 'health settings'. About one in five of social workers and front line managers employed by Social Services Departments in England and Wales work in hospitals or community health centres. Of these about 95 per cent are based in hospitals (Social Services Inspectorate 1993). Research into the effectiveness of hospital social work has demonstrated, in line with evidence from the United States (Bywaters 1990), that social workers can positively influence the quality of patients' experience of hospital, make 'discharge planning' more effective and raise the level and quality of services provided after discharge. As a result, the likelihood of readmission through the resurgence of ill health is reduced. (See Connor and Tibbitt 1988; McLeod 1994a; Russell 1989; Townsend *et al.* 1988).

Studies of the relatively small number of social worker attachments to General Practice centres also indicate that take-up of financial benefits, counselling and home care services is boosted in populations previously unknown to social services. Feedback from the users concerned has identified this as crucial to averting the collapse of independent living and much attendant suffering (Cumella 1994; Ruddy 1992).

The crux of such practice is that social work intervention can temper inclement social conditions which are associated with poor health. This has two important implications. First, social work practice generally, not only in health settings, has the potential to be health work, i.e., to contribute to the promotion of good health, the prevention or treatment of illness, or the care of people who are living with ill health (Bywaters 1993). Second, inasmuch as social work intervention increases users' personal and material resources, it may act as a counterweight to the detrimental effects on health associated with social incqualities.

However, social work practice does not necessarily result in a more equitable experience of health. To give three examples: social workers operate within a policy framework which may conflict with reducing inequality; social workers are unlikely to be free from discriminatory attitudes and work in discriminatory systems; and inadequate resources may inhibit the development of approaches which might be more equitable.

Social workers are key figures in the assessment and care management approach at the centre of current arrangements for community care established by the NHS and Community Care Act, 1990 (Department of Health 1992a). Whilst exhorted to enhance independence, increase choice, support carers and provide services sensitive to the needs of ethnic minorities (Department of Health 1989), social workers are required to operate within a market-based economy of care designed to provide control over state expenditure (and to favour the private sector). Within such a system, equity is not an objective. So, for example, social workers are engaged in assessing older people's eligibility for means-tested residential or community care, against a backdrop of the rapid withdrawal of provision for free long-stay health care (Henwood 1992). The greater reliance on informal carers is certain to increase the unequal balance of care work done by women, with overall negative consequences for their physical and emotional health both while caring and subsequently (Graham 1993).

Similarly, the proposal that a market-led approach will respond to the needs of minority groups is based on questionable assumptions. It requires both that the needs of minority groups are as likely to be identified as those of the majority and that there are no barriers to establishing appropriate provision. Neither assumption holds good.

Despite an emphasis on 'anti-discriminatory' practice in social work training (Central Council for Education and Training in Social Work – CCETSW – 1989), there is continuing evidence from surveys of disabled users' experience, that misinformation and prejudice, as well as the embedded nature of institutional oppression, are pervasive. Hence, there is no guarantee that needs will be assessed even-handedly (Morris 1993). The development of private domiciliary and residential care provision depends, amongst other things, on the availability of capital for investment. Inequitable access to capital is reflected in the continuing dearth of private sector provision geared to members of ethnic minority groups. Black elders are commonly faced with no appropriate alternative to the scattered examples of small scale, self-help initiatives funded on a short-term basis which cater for their specific requirements (Patel 1993).

The inadequate resources allocated to social services have also been shown to undermine attempts to develop more equal and participatory provision. Neill and Williams' (1992) study of older patients discharged from hospital showed that pre-discharge, hospital social workers did participate in inter-professional reviews of patients' home circumstances. However, staffing levels were such that one out of three patients did not have the opportunity to discuss how they would manage at home and, when interviewed after discharge, two-thirds were found to be experiencing difficulty with self-care tasks, most still felt unwell and in some degree of pain, while about one third were assessed as possibly depressed.

Despite these negative tendencies, there are signs of a growing determination to tackle the impact of social inequalities on health through social work (Auluck and Iles 1991; Bywaters 1986; 1993; Cemlyn 1993; Holman 1991; McLeod 1994a; Patel 1993; Scrutton 1992; Sheppard 1991). Three diverse examples of this trend will be discussed in this chapter. First, an initiative in a 'health setting' concerning older people's access to a Social Services Department's hospital-based services; second, an example of local authority practice not in a 'health setting' but with implications for health: the beginnings of policy and practice developments to combat the impact of inequality on the health of young people in residential care; and, third, locality-based group work with women to secure less stigmatizing approaches to health care.

While local and incremental gains have resulted from these projects, they also reveal that a significant shift in health experience requires more fundamental changes in social and economic relations.

Health related social work emerges as needing to contribute to, and be underwritten by, initiatives which have such profound changes as their objective.

Improving access to health resources for older patients

This project aimed to improve older patients' access to hospital social work services as crucial resources for health by encouraging self-referral. It was based in an 'acute elderly unit' for patients aged seventy-five or over in a district general hospital.

Previous research had indicated that, despite the benefits for older patients' health arising from access to hospital social work services (Connor and Tibbitt 1988; Neill and Williams 1992; Russell 1989; Townsend *et al.* 1988), rates of self-referral for hospital social work were consistently low (Social Services Inspectorate 1992; 1993). This hospital reflected the common pattern. Patients were usually referred when medical professionals – predominantly doctors or nurses – decided it was appropriate, passing on the request through inter-professional ward meetings. Evidence from other studies indicated that this approach does not identify all patients who would benefit from referral (Bywaters 1991; Neill and Williams 1992) and, in a situation of shortage of resources, tends to be used by social workers as a buffer to the increased demands for services that encouraging self-referral would bring (McLeod 1994a).

The preliminary stage of the project had demonstrated that most older patients – 73 per cent – were unaware of the existence of hospital social workers and could not identify accurately what they could provide. Moreover, although the most serious cases of immediate risk had been picked up, on average 14 per cent of patients each week required social work intervention but were not referred. Some of these patients seemed to be wrestling with social conditions which caused a great deal of suffering and threatened future deterioration in health. In addition, the circumstances of some patients needed checking by a social worker because they could not be assumed to be safe or unproblematic, notably in the case of patients who were already disadvantaged through sensory or cognitive impairment or whose first language was not English (McLeod 1994a).

The project now aimed to promote self-referral by ensuring older patients were better informed about hospital social work and by addressing disadvantage amongst older patients. The main features and outcome of the approach are summarized here. (For a more detailed account see McLeod 1994b). A specially designed leaflet was produced explaining the existence of the service and what it could offer. It was translated into Punjabi, Hindi and Urdu, the most common first languages other than English in the area, and stated that an interpreting service could be available. A large print version and a cassette recording were made. The leaflet also stated the Department's commitment to services for gay and lesbian people.

Over six weeks, hospital social workers briefly introduced themselves to all newly admitted patients, gave out the leaflet, explained what was available and made it clear how they could be contacted. Where patients had a severe degree of cognitive impairment their carers were briefed as well. Seventy-six patients out of the total of eighty-seven admissions were contacted. ·

Now, when interviewed, 64 per cent of patients knew of the service and 56 per cent could describe accurately what social workers did. The outcome was a substantial increase in the rate of self-referral – eleven across the six-week period of the project compared to two in the previous six months. A doubling of the usual rate of referrals to the key worker indicated that the approach had reached new populations. Patients who self-referred requested social work help appropriately, i.e., they required packages of care ranging from simple to complex. This offers further confirmation that it is in older patients' interests to gain access to the means of referral for hospital social work.

Combining the leaflet with personal contact was beneficial, the main sources of information cited being initial contact with a social worker and the leaflet. About 50 per cent of patients commented positively on the usefulness of the leaflet; however, the crucial importance of introductory personal contact was demonstrated by ten out of the eleven self-referrals occurring immediately at that point.

The effectiveness of the project in meeting patients' diverse requirements was variable. Analysis revealed that over 50 per cent of patients had sensory, cognitive and/or physical impairments. Team members concluded that services based on an assumption that communication problems were a 'special need' needed to change to services based on a recognition that this was the norm, for example, by routinely printing the leaflet in larger print and production of the cassette in Hindi, Urdu and Punjabi.

In a situation of rapid turnover of patients and high pressure on staff there was continued evidence of institutionalized discrimination against disabled people and members of ethnic minorities:

interpreting services were not accessed routinely and, where patients were profoundly cognitively impaired, social workers still did not routinely check with a carer whether there was a need for social work intervention.

The project produced increased job satisfaction. Team members had enjoyed the personal contacts devoted to briefing patients and found they had been able to operate more effectively in ward meetings because they already knew who patients were. However, the project also demonstrated that opening up self-referral led to increased workload demands. The referral rate doubled, the key worker estimated working an extra half day per week.

Discussion

The project demonstrated the benefits of promoting access to resources by recognizing older patients' own expertise in assessing their requirements and by addressing disadvantage amongst them. However, as with Social Services Departments generally, this particular Department was underfunded for community care measures (Hoyes *et al.* 1994). This meant that no extra staffing resources were forthcoming to assist with the doubled rate of referral and the staff time allocated for initial contacts. Therefore, the new approach was unlikely to be sustainable. Hence the project exposed that attempts to improve access are ultimately constrained by the trend against redistributing material resources to older people, the majority of whom live within or on the margins of poverty (Walker 1990).

It may be that even if the new approach to referral in the project setting does not last long, it will still amount to a degree of counter pressure against prevailing social inequalities in the interests of older people's health. First, it will provide more systematic evidence of need, a necessary foundation for making a case for such needs to be met. Second, workers may come to have a more substantial investment in this way of working. Third, a small, but nevertheless greater, number of patients and carers will know who to ask for help and therefore have an investment in this sort of help being available.

However, these potentially positive outcomes of hospital social workers' attempts to construct a more egalitarian experience of health care for older people serve to highlight the need for more fundamental changes in resource distribution, in favour of older people, on a national scale and, as integral to this, the legitimation of access to such resources as a right.

Sexual health policy and practice

The second example centres on the development of initiatives to combat the impact of inequality on the sexual health of young people in residential care. Drawing on discussions with specialist workers holding particular responsibilities for this aspect of practice, this focuses on emerging policies and practices covering issues of sexuality in three Social Services Departments.

The emergence of AIDS over the past fifteen years has had the effect of pushing sexuality up the public health agenda to become one of the five target areas for *The Health of the Nation* (Department of Health 1992b). The language in which it is discussed, as 'sexual health', and the focus of attention, on HIV transmission and teenage pregnancy, reflect a perspective which centres on concepts of risk and dangerousness rather than on the difficulties of securing rights in an unequal society.

This focus can also be seen in the growing body of research about risks associated with sexuality faced by young people living in residential care, including abuse, pregnancy and involvement in prostitution (Garnett 1992; Katz and Brindle 1991; Sobsey 1994).

Emerging from the social workers' practice was evidence that these risks are compounded by inequalities associated with the young people's residential status. Such young people may experience:

- reduced opportunities to learn about and explore sexuality. Whilst peers rather than adults may be the major source of learning about sex for most young people, residents may have less access to information through missing sex education lessons at school, reduced skills and confidence in reading and, lacking continuity in relationships, less opportunities for conversation with significant adults. They may also have less privacy to learn about sex from videos, reading or experimentation;
- difficulties in asserting rights or making informed choices about sexual relationships, and in accessing relevant public services (e.g. family planning, advice or medical services). The stigma of being 'in care' may exacerbate a limited sense of personal control and lowered self-esteem;
- institutionalized homophobia and racism in the care system (Community Care Inside 1994). Examples from these Departments included homophobic attitudes and behaviour by staff and by fellow residents. Restricted opportunities for information, discussion and experimentation are far more pronounced for young gay

and lesbian people whose identity may be strongly disapproved of and for whom sexual expression may be illegal (Brindle 1994). Myths about Black people's sexuality are still prevalent (Baxter 1994) and young Black residents are less likely than their White counterparts to have adults amongst the staff with whom they might identify and, perhaps, in whom they might feel able to confide; and

• unequal treatment from staff between or within residential units. In the absence of clear guidance, training and support, staff inevitably rely on their own, varied, values (Bremner and Hillin 1991). These inequalities arise, in part, because of an uncertainty amongst staff about whether sexual information and expression is a right to be encouraged or a risk to be avoided.

The three Departments' responses to issues of sexuality for young residents can be seen to reflect attempts to combat these inequalities, particularly through raising consciousness. First, parallel to moving beyond a 'colour-blind' approach in combating racism, a central plank of the developing strategy on sexuality in these Departments is to make the issues *visible* through discussion and training while creating *legitimacy* within the agency through the establishment of formal policies approved by senior managers and Councillors. In one agency an increased reporting by residential staff of concerns about sexual abuse has followed this approach.

Second, explicitly offering information and discussion to young people in residential care, through small group work and statutory review processes, is intended to help develop a climate of rights and openness rather than secrecy and dependency (Katz and Brindle 1991). In addition, establishing and publicizing complaints procedures aims to redress the powerlessness felt by young people in residential care.

Third, working with both parents and with other agencies is designed to promote more open knowledge and discussion of sexuality in a wider context. Examples of this approach include the distribution of leaflets explaining policies to parents, the establishment of a joint funded advice centre aimed at young people and work between Social Services and Education Departments to provide information and education through schools and youth clubs.

However, the Departments studied also differed in the emphasis placed on inequality and rights rather than personal risks. For example, attitudes to gay and lesbian residents varied. One authority explicitly stated its opposition to Section 28 of the Local Government Act 1988 as 'discriminatory' while another covered the issue of same-sex relationships in a phrase about 'acceptance, respect and support for individuals' sexual expression and identity'. There were also differences in the focus of the education given to young people. In one agency it was strongly felt that information which emphasized risks would not be absorbed by young people who wanted to know how to have 'good' sex, not just be told what not to do by adults who had a wider range of opportunities.

Discussion

While these local authority initiatives have some important possibilities for combating inequalities, they operate in the context of central government policies which undermine efforts to develop equality in sexual health. The continuing scapegoating of single parents and young mothers, attacks on sex education in schools and the withdrawal of approval for a sex education guide aimed at young people are three recent examples of the Government's overall approach (Brown and Wynn Davies 1993; Hunt 1994; Pithers 1994). In one of the authorities studied, a specific consequence was a delay in the production of a play with a sex education message to be presented in schools. A wider indirect consequence is to create uncertainties which encourage authorities and individual workers to continue to leave sexual issues hidden.

Second, this ambivalence about sexual rights in general, and gay and lesbian sexuality in particular, is reflected in the muddled framework of legislation under which social workers have to operate. The differential age of consent for young gay men, compared to lesbian women or heterosexual couples, means that they are less likely to have access to safe environments in which to meet other gay men and develop relationships and even less likely to come out to social workers or other responsible adults (Wynn Davies *et al.* 1994). The clause in the 1956 Sexual Offences Act which makes it illegal for 'defectives' to have sexual relationships outside marriage obstructs the development of sexual health work with young people with learning disabilities.

Third, as with smoking (Graham 1987), the material circumstances in which choices about health are made can be seen to have a crucial effect. One consequence of Government policy over the past fifteen years has been to raise the age at which the majority of young people enter the labour market, while making them more dependent on their parents for housing and income. The relatively young age at which people 'in care' are expected to live 'independently' and the limited support provided by social services or housing authorities and the social security system, create difficult choices about how to obtain money. For young care leavers who are homeless or isolated and perhaps have already been sexually abused, the choice to earn by selling sexual 'favours' may be a realistic response to material difficulties which themselves are damaging to health (Boseley 1994; Char 1994; Community Care 1994).

Fourth, the drive towards the privatization of health and welfare provision has resulted in a larger number of agencies and companies being involved in the purchasing and providing of health, education and social care. This is proving a further obstacle to attempts to develop strategic responses to health issues, including sexual health.

Social Services Departments' developing policies on 'sexual health' for young people 'in care' can have some impact on redressing the inequalities they face but are ultimately dependent on more equitable government policies relating to social security, housing and employment opportunities as well as directly to sexuality.

Women's health: a groupwork initiative[1]

The catalyst for practice here was a community worker's self-criticism and commitment to democratizing health education:

> Initially I found it hard to raise and promote health issues locally – workshops and talks attracted small groups that listened and went home. This was despite researching topics of interest, appropriate times and providing childcare support.
>
> I needed to discover more about local women's feelings and experiences of health care before I could start to look at experts coming in to 'educate' in a way that was putting more pressure on people often already under stress, directly or indirectly, as a result of living in a low income area.
>
> I also felt that the views of women on estates like the Heath are less well known than the views of more middle class communities, so that it would be productive to encourage women to record their feelings and experiences in booklet form.
>
> (O'Hora 1994)

This led to a range of initiatives, three of which are discussed here:

1 action to shape local General Practitioners' (GPs') practices more in residents' interests;
2 a head lice campaign to lessen stigmatization and increase access to useful health care resources; and
3 the use of publications as campaigning tools locally and to develop more widespread recognition of the undermining effects of poverty on health.

GP practice

Women who were already Adult Basic Education students at a local community centre, and others who might be interested, were approached to work in a small group producing accounts of their experiences of health care.

Initially the group looked at their experiences of GPs and role-played various scenarios. Several consistent themes of dissatisfaction emerged:

• the feeling of being quickly labelled an over-protective or irresponsible mother;
• unsympathetic responses from receptionists when least able to deal with this;
• lack of play areas for children;
• timing of surgeries; and
• inadequate explanations from GPs.

The group invited local GPs to discuss these issues. A GP from one partnership responded. She confirmed that receptionists should never refuse appointments, asserted that patients must insist on proper explanations from their doctor and was responsive to the request for early evening surgeries to accommodate the needs of people who could not afford, or risk, taking time off from work. Her Practice subsequently acted on these issues.

Later the women commented that they had felt able to express views and feelings that would have been impossible to convey individually. In turn, the doctors from this surgery attended the launch of the women's booklet (which will be discussed later) and made copies available in their waiting rooms. They also continued to meet periodically with the group. The main lesson from this initiative was the possibility of shifting existing power imbalances which limit the effectiveness of health care, through developing informed, collective pressure groups.

Head lice campaign

The group also identified common concerns about the head lice situation locally and decided to hold an open meeting on the subject, inviting the secretary of the local Community Health Council (CHC).

About thirty local mothers came, through word of mouth alone. There was anger and frustration over the very high level of head lice infestation and that school nurses no longer checked children's hair. There was also great confusion over treatment and annoyance at the difficulty of obtaining the lotion for this, while certain local families were scapegoated for spreading the infestation. As a result, the CHC secretary organized another meeting between the doctor in charge of public health, four members of the women's group, two head teachers, the community worker and the Director of Nursing Services.

Over a series of meetings this committee sorted out several difficulties:

- many of the myths about head lice were exploded, for example, that 'dirty families have them';
- the roles of parents, teachers and nurses were clarified;
- a clinic providing lotion was established nearby – previously it had been at some distance from the estate; and
- a Health Authority leaflet on head lice issued through schools was rewritten and redesigned by the Adult Basic Education Unit, as many parents could not understand the original.

A questionnaire by the Women's Group revealed that 75 per cent of parents did not know their children's school nurse, 50 per cent did not know how to contact her and 50 per cent did not know how to get to the centre where nurses were based. The Nursing Director responded by increasing publicity and ensuring there was some regularity in nurses' availability in schools.

The local community worker rated the efforts of the local women committee members – as health workers – very highly.

They worked very hard at disseminating information – discussions in shops and àt the school gates were common. They are still approached by neighbours and friends wanting help on a variety of health issues as they are seen as able to get things done and having an understanding of how things work. Judging by what is generally said about head lice in the area now, the four women were far more effective educators than the Health Authority experts or myself.

(O'Hora 1994)

This action illustrates the possibility of changing health prevention and treatment measures from forms of stigmatizing policing to opportunities for self-control on the part of local populations. It also illustrates the importance of doing so if uptake is to be increased.

Publications

Besides helping to develop a collective consciousness of problems and acting as a focus for action, production of the booklet, 'Don't Ask Us We're Just The Patients', enhanced the group's confidence. They compiled it from brief accounts of their experience of health and health care. As described in a subsequent resumé of their work:

> The title of the book was chosen by the group as it seemed to spell out everything we all wanted to say. The book proved to be a tremendous success and has made many G.P.s sit up and take notice and some practices have altered since the publication.

The booklet is an educational resource. Accounts not only provide useful feedback about being on the receiving end of medical examination, they also bring home from first hand experience the effects on women's health of working and parenting in relative poverty (Graham 1993).

> In the day I am a dinner lady and at night I am a cleaner. . . . I have four children. . . . When school ends, I go home, prepare the dinner and then go out to work. When I get home from work, I sit with the children and we read books. Then I bath two of them and put them to bed . . . I have to do all this with two jobs because we cannot manage on my husband's wages alone. The rent, gas, and electricity bills take up most of the money I earn and my husband's wages pay for clothes and the car so my life is very active . . . I have to carry on just to survive. But saying that I need a break just to wind down.

The group also drew on a professional research survey, 'The Extent of Credit and Debt', sponsored by the city and county councils and based on 245 households in the area. The survey's findings were used as a basis for applications for funding. Reference to the survey also contributed to drawing attention to the general case for viewing low income as having a critical effect on health and well-being and to evidence on the need for national policies to increase benefit levels. For example, the survey report described how more than half the households were dependent on welfare benefits or a state pension.

> A quarter of all respondents said that they could only afford to keep one room of their home warm and one in twenty that they could not afford to keep any of their home warm. Families with children were more likely to say this than older people.

Discussion

While having their greatest impact locally, the initiatives of the women's health group provide certain central lessons. 'Health education' of professionals can result in them making common cause with lay health workers in developments leading to more equitable and effective experiences of health services. Once provided with the resources to develop collective action to challenge health inequalities, populations which might otherwise tend to be scapegoated as undermining their own health through 'unwise health behaviours' can identify and work towards establishing social conditions with major benefits for health – not only for themselves but more generally.

CONCLUSION – DELIVERING ON HEALTH

All three sets of initiatives demonstrate that attempts to tackle the impact of social inequalities on health are starting to develop as an integral part of social work practice. Some lessons emerge: for example, the significance of impairment as an additional source of disadvantage amongst older hospital patients, the importance of recognizing sexuality as an issue of inequality and not just of individual risk and the need for the health education of professionals by lay people as well as vice versa. At every stage achievements rested on the quality of working relations with others outside social work – patients, users, residents, other health professionals, policy makers. The vulnerability of such initiatives is also apparent: the financial context was one of short-term local and central government funding, cut backs, low priority and marginal rather than mainstream status. However, in each case local gains were achieved by very different forms of practice.

Despite their success, these initiatives also demonstrate a central limitation of social work which cannot secure the major shifts in the distribution of material resources or have the broad ranging impact on discrimination which is needed to significantly improve the health of the population. Social work's contribution is necessarily incremental, achieved through alliances with both lay and professional health workers.

NOTES

1 We should like to acknowledge the work of Sue Boulter, Jan Headley, Sue Houlton, Pam Kelb, Ruth O'Hora and Hazel Williamson in preparing this section.

REFERENCES

Auluck, R. and Iles, P. (1991) 'The Referral Process: A Study of Working Relationships Between Ante-natal Clinic Nursing Staff and Hospital Social Workers and their Impact on Asian Women', *British Journal of Social Work* 21 (1): 41–62.

Baxter, C. (1994) 'Sex Education in the Multi-racial Society', in Craft, A. (ed.) *Practice Issues in Sexuality and Learning Difficulties*, London: Routledge.

Boseley, S. (1994) 'Runaway Children "Cut off from carers"', *Guardian*, 23 November: 2.

Bremner, J. and Hillin, A. (1991) *Sexuality, Young People and Care*, London: CCETSW.

Brindle, D. (1994) 'Birmingham May Register Care Home For Gay Children', *Guardian*, 15 July: 5.

Brown, C. and Wynn Davies, P. (1993) 'Single Parents Targeted For Welfare Cuts', *Independent* 6 October: 8.

Bywaters, P. (1986) 'Social Work and The Medical Profession: Arguments Against Unconditional Collaboration', *British Journal of Social Work* 16: 661–77.

—— (1990) 'Discharge Planning – The American Experience', unpublished, Coventry University: Department of Applied Social Studies.

—— (1991) 'Casefinding and Screening For Social Work in Acute General Hospitals', *British Journal of Social Work* 21 (1): 19–40.

—— (1993) 'Social Work – Health Work', *Practice* 6 (4): 277–84.

CCETSW (1989) *Dip SW Requirements and Regulations For The Diploma In Social Work; Paper 30*, London: CCETSW.

Cemlyn, S. (1993) 'Health and Social Work: Working With Gypsies and Travellers', *Practice* 6 (4): 246–61.

Char (1994) *Acting in Isolation*, London: Char.

Clare, A.W. and Corney, R. (eds) (1982) *Social Work and Primary Health Care*, London: Academic Press.

Community Care (1994) 'The Price of Independence', *Community Care* 1–7 September: 12–13.

Community Care Inside (1994) 'Anti-discriminatory Practice', *Community Care* 31 March.

Connor, A. and Tibbitt, J. (1988) *Social Workers and Health Care In Hospitals*, Edinburgh: HMSO.

Cumella, S. (1994) *Care Management In A Primary Healthcare Team*, University of Birmingham: Centre for Research and Information into Mental Disability.

Department of Health (1989) *Caring for People*, London: HMSO.

—— (1992a) *Assessment and Care Management: A Practitioners Guide*, London: HMSO.

—— (1992b) *The Health of the Nation: A Strategy for Health in England*, London: HMSO.

Garnett, L. (1992) *Leaving Care and After*, London: National Children's Bureau.

Graham, H. (1987) 'Women's Smoking and Family Health', *Social Science and Medicine* 25 (1): 47–56.

—— (1993) *Hardship and Health in Women's Lives*, London: Harvester Wheatsheaf.

Henwood, M. (1992) *Through a Glass Darkly: Community Care and Elderly People*, London: King's Fund Institute.

Holman, B. (1991) 'It's No Accident', *Poverty* 80: 6–8.

Hoyes, L., Lart, R., Means, R. and Taylor, M. (1994) *Community Care in Transition*, York: Joseph Rowntree Trust.

Hunt, L. (1994) 'Sex Education Curbs Will Mean More Pregnancies', *Independent*, 30 March: 2.

Katz, I. and Brindle, D. (1991) 'Child Care Head Gets Life Terms', *Guardian*, 30 November: 1.

McLeod, E. (1994a) 'Patients in Inter-professional Practice', in Soothill, K., Mackay, L. and Webb, C. (eds) *Interprofessional Issues in Health Care*, London: Edward Arnold.

—— (1994b) 'Older Patients and Access to Hospital Social Work: Boosting Self-referral', unpublished, University of Warwick.

Morris, J. (1993) 'Feminism and Disability', *Feminist Review* 43, Spring: 57–70.

Neill, J. and Williams, J. (1992) *Leaving Hospital*, London: National Institute for Social Work.

O'Hora, R. (1994) Personal communication.

Patel, N. (1993) 'Healthy Margins: Black Elders' Care – Models, Policies and Prospects', in Ahmad, W.I.U. (ed.) *'Race' and Health in Contemporary Britain*, Milton Keynes: Open University Press.

Pithers, M. (1994) '"Smutty" Booklet is Withdrawn From Shops', *Independent*, 24 March: 3.

Ruddy, B. (1992) 'Brief Encounters', *Health Service Journal*, 17 September: 22–4.

Russell, J. (1989) *South Glamorgan Care For The Elderly Hospital Discharge Service*, University of Cardiff: School of Social and Administrative Studies.

Scrutton, S. (1992) *Ageing, Healthy and In Control*, London: Chapman and Hall.

Shaw, A. (1991) *Review of Health-Based Social Work in Avon*, Bristol: Avon Social Services Department.

Sheppard, M. (1991) 'General Practice, Social Work, and Mental Health Sections: The Social Control of Women', *British Journal of Social Work* 21 (6): 663–84.

Sobsey, D. (1994) 'Sexual Abuse of Individuals with Intellectual Disability', in Craft, A. (ed.) *Practice Issues in Sexuality and Learning Difficulties*, London: Routledge.

Social Services Inspectorate (1992) *An Inspection of Social Work in General Hospitals*, Belfast: Social Services Inspectorate, Department of Health and Social Security.

—— (1993) *Social Services For Hospital Patients 1: Working At The Interface*, London: Department of Health.

Townsend, J., Piper, M., Frank, A.O., Dyer, S., North, W.R.S. and Meade, T.W. (1988) 'Reduction in Hospital Readmission Stay Of Elderly Patients By A Community Based Discharge Scheme: A Randomised Controlled Trial', *British Medical Journal* 297: 544–47.

Walker, A. (1990) 'The Benefits of Old Age? Age Discrimination and Social Security', in McEwen, E. (ed.) *Age: The Unrecognised Discrimination*, London: Age Concern.

Wynn Davies, P., Brown, C. and Macdonald, M. (1994) 'Sexual Equality For Gays Rejected', *Independent*, 2 February: 1.

Chapter 5

Caught in the caring trap

The health of children who care

Jo Aldridge and Saul Becker

INTRODUCTION

Since the 1960s much has been written about the effects of parental illness or disability on the development of children. However, until recently very little attention has focused on the impact on children of caring for their own disabled parents, providing for their domestic, social and personal welfare and taking on responsibilities that are usually associated with adulthood.

Discussion of the effects of parental illness or disability in public debate has tended to highlight health issues in relation to parental care of children, especially the stresses and strains involved in having to cope with the presence of illness (or disability) in the family; the cognitive implications (the extent and nature of children's understanding of illness/disability); role model diversification; changes in familial relations; social stigma; and even the revision of physical activities and recreation with the family (see Anthony 1970; Beard 1975). However, our evidence suggests that where children are also carers a new framework of variables must be addressed. When examining the impact of caring on children we must consider not only all the aforementioned issues of having to deal with the presence of parental illness or disability, but also, and perhaps more significantly, the impact on children of the caring *commitment*. When children are carers, we have to consider their quality of life; their ability to participate in social intercourse; their opportunities to interact with their peers; their educational attainments; their access to a life beyond the often restricted, home-bound experiences of caring; and the impact of privation, injustice and inequality brought about by the neglect of welfare services. In this chapter we demonstrate how these children are caught in a 'caring trap' because of their dual role as children *and* as carers. We discuss how under such conditions children experience the most profound inequities, the most acute neglect, with major implications for their own health and well-being. Finally, we consider initiatives which would begin to meet children's right to be treated equitably, and with respect, as carers.

THE IDENTITY OF YOUNG CARERS

We define children who care as those children/young people under the age of eighteen whose lives are restricted by caring for a sick or disabled person in the home. Relatively little is known about the number of young carers in the UK although early small scale surveys estimated that there could be 10, 000 children who are carrying out caring duties (O'Neill 1988; Page 1988). However, it is likely that this figure is a gross underestimation. The 1990 General Household Survey of Carers calculated that approximately 6.8 million people aged sixteen or over in Great Britain were looking after a sick, disabled or older person (Office of Population Censuses and Surveys 1992). Much of this and other 'informal' care is carried out by children, but it is impossible to derive accurate figures of the scope.

However, there is an argument to suggest that, presently at least, the pursuit of detailed statistics in this respect would prove relatively unproductive (Aldridge and Becker 1993a). It is now widely documented that children undertake major caring responsibilities in the home (see Bilsborrow 1992; Meredith 1991; 1992) and that they have done so for many years (Aldridge and Becker 1993a). Children undertake these tasks in a largely secretive or covert manner because of the fears associated with caring, in particular of the consequences of coming to the attention of welfare professionals. Until these fears are addressed, and allayed, by health professionals, social workers and educationalists alike, it will be very difficult to generate any accurate assessment of the numbers, characteristics and location of young carers.

Against this background, our chapter is also unable to offer detailed evidence of the ways in which inequalities between young carers and adult carers, on the one hand, and young carers and other children, on the other, are compounded by factors of class, gender, 'race' and, indeed, disability or poor health amongst the child carers themselves. Evidence from studies of adult informal carers makes clear the significance of these factors. The increasing influence of wealth and income in securing social care, the gendered bias in 'selection' for caring and in the support received from informal and public services, the persistence of myths concerning Black families 'looking after their own' which result in reduced services, the continuing failure of services to be responsive to a wide range of needs and the evidence that professionals contribute to the disabling of people living with physical impairments are all examples of factors which are unlikely to be irrelevant when the carers are under eighteen (Biggs 1987; Morris 1993; Patel 1993; Ungerson 1987).

THE NATURE AND CONSEQUENCES OF CARING

From our research into the experiences and needs of young carers and their families (Aldridge and Becker 1993a; 1994a), it was clear that these children were facing many problems and difficulties: caring restricted their lives as children; and, as care providers, they were at best undervalued and at worst excluded, denied access to services and provision available to adult carers. We have characterized this as being *punished* for caring (Aldridge and Becker 1993b). These children were, and continue to be, overlooked by professionals across a range of disciplines and sectors and neglected by family, friends and the local community.

The tasks of caring

Young carers are performing a wide range of tasks from basic domestic duties to very private or intimate 'nursing' responsibilities such as bathing, dressing and toileting their parent/s. The complexion and intensity of tasks carried out by young carers clearly depends on the nature and extent of their parent's needs, as well as the availability of support either from within the family unit or externally from professional carers.

Although *some* young carers' duties may be considered to be the same as those expected of any child from a 'regular' household in which disability or long-term illness is not present and where children do not have to take on caring responsibilities, certain tasks would be widely acknowledged as unacceptable for children to be undertaking. The World Health Organization (1982) identified the adoption of responsibility in the home as a specific need in terms of a child's development. However, it emphasized the 'gradual' extension of responsibility, an onus concurrent with the child's age and which coincided with their graduated progression into maturity. For many carers the passage into caring and responsibility is neither gradual nor concomitant with age. It is not a rite of passage into the adult arena, but a sudden claim on their time and energies which constricts, and concludes, their childhood.

Working out what is acceptable in terms of children's caring responsibilities is not easy. Should a child of, say, twelve or thirteen be undertaking duties that include lifting their parent onto the toilet, washing and dressing them, with all the potential hazards and problems that this may bring? Not only could there be physical consequences of a child carrying out such tasks (such as injury to either child or care receiver), but we must also consider the possible psychological effects on children of having to proffer intimate care provision for their parent. For example, washing, dressing and toileting a parent is not a conventional facet of familial relations. As one of our young carers said: 'I was having to take my dad to the toilet, clean him up when he couldn't get to the toilet . . . no one should have to see their parents like that' (Aldridge and Becker 1993a: vi).

Thus, when considering the acceptable or unacceptable face of child caring, respect must be paid to the feelings and wishes of both the parents and their child carers, *including* the acknowledgement of such issues as the embarrassment or possible humiliation involved in the experience of children caring. From our studies it was clear that neither children nor parents were comfortable with the intimate nursing role children were often forced to adopt in the home, but neither party wanted child caring duties to cease altogether. It is a sad fact that, presently at least, there are few schemes in place that can acknowledge and resolve this caring dilemma.

An obligatory role

For many young carers the caring role is obligatory within the family. They are not consulted or given the chance to resist or deny the adoption of the caring role. Although this may seem improbable, it was clear from our studies that in many instances the caring role is forced on children by other more dominant individuals either in the family or outside (professionals who substitute their support for that of a young child). We found evidence of fathers or siblings who would select a younger, less dominant member of the family to take on the care they would not or could not do themselves. In most other cases children were left with little choice but to undertake caring as the onset of illness or disability in the family often irrevocably transformed the family unit. That is, when the illness or disability was first diagnosed the able parent left the family home and the care of the disabled or long-term sick parent was left in the hands of their child (in most cases it was the father who left and refused to provide care).

Caring alone

Not only is the caring role obligatory, many young carers are also left to cope alone. Outside the immediate family, members of the extended family, neighbours and friends seemed to persistently deny their support. Furthermore, professional caring support (community care assistants, nurses etc.) focused almost exclusively on the needs of the ill/disabled parent, even though these professionals regularly worked within the family unit where children were caring. Many professionals who could have identified young carers through their contact with families were failing to do so. In many cases this was simply because they were unaware of the issue itself or had found no direct evidence of care management by children in the home. However, such neglect by professionals in some cases could not simply be explained through oversight.

We found evidence of three characteristic responses by professionals:

- **Unintentional silence**   (professionals were aware of child caring but did not know how to help and so did nothing to support child carers); or
- **Intentional conspiracy**   (they knew the child was caring, did not offer help but colluded in exploiting their caring labours by withdrawing their own support and allowing the child carer to take up the shortfall). We encountered professionals who were not only aware of young carers in families, but also blatantly exploited their labours either as a supplement to their own care provision or sometimes as a substitute for it. For example, we found several examples of community care assistance being withdrawn from families where children were caring because the child carers were considered 'old enough' to care. The age criterion applied by community care assistants ranged from twelve to sixteen. Some professionals simply withdrew their support arbitrarily:

> My mum asked if the home help could give her a shower and she told her there was no point in her coming as she had two daughters who could help. They said 'we only come to the people who need our help'. Sarah, fifteen, a young carer.
>
> (Aldridge and Becker 1993a: 38)

This inequitable situation was compounded by the fear child carers had of coming to the attention of professionals who, to both children and parents alike, represented a threat – of separation and the dissolution of caring and family ties – which meant the existence of care provision by children was kept hidden and private within the family. There is evidence to suggest that this fear experienced by child carers and their parents is not unfounded; that the separation of families is an all too common response (see Meredith 1991). To some extent young carers' fear of welfare services serves to reinforce their invisibility from professionals and their powerlessness as carers (they are reluctant, because of their fear, to seek help) and as children – as Alderson (1992: 163) says, 'children are the least powerful social group'.

Disadvantageous consequences

The consequences of caring involved a series of further disadvantages which carried profound penalties for children's well-being.

The impact of caring on children's lives outside the caring (home) environment where relatives and professional carers alike continually overlooked their needs, was profound and potentially far-reaching. For many young carers, school life was both problematic and fragmentary. Understandably, most young carers found it difficult to reconcile the world of caring with school life. The commitment they gave to caring often made them late, and erratic attendance patterns and long-term absences were a common feature of child caring (as a consequence, under-achievement was also common). Such patterns were maintained and even reinforced by the attitude and approaches of teachers or educationalists who were failing to identify young carers at school (they were guilty of *unintentionally neglecting* young carers). When such professionals did recognize child carers they were either unable to provide solutions, offered inappropriate responses or chose to disbelieve children's caring accounts – their response was *unintentionally silent* (see Aldridge and Becker 1993a).

The extent of the commitment children give to caring often also meant they had little access to peer group friendships and recreation. Children who did not have to physically care for their parents could neither easily relate to the concept of caring in this way nor to the impact and effects of caring. A consequence of caring was that young carers engaged in very unpredictable friendship patterns due to the time and attention given over to caring duties, their lack of school attendance (where traditionally many peer friendships are formed and develop), their inability to participate fully in social activities, the stigma associated with illness or disability (or drug/alcohol abuse) and the lack of home space and time in which to conduct friendships. Thus, peer friendships – already balancing on shifting sands when caring interceded – became disparate and constrained and could eventually cease altogether, further reinforcing the isolation and exclusion that is commonly the young caring experience.

A further dimension to the inequity children experience as carers was that as well as being largely unrecognized, their caring labours were unpaid. Furthermore, the dedication they gave to their caring role undermined their opportunities to gain part-time work (age permitting). They were part of a caring world that was mostly hidden and which operated in an arena of poverty, powerlessness and exclusion. By being denied access to paid work they were denied any sense of the independence or self-esteem that a personal income, no matter how small, might have provided.

Furthermore, remuneration was unlikely to come from other sources as the social security system does not support young carers either. They are neither eligible for the Carers Premium nor can they apply for social fund payments. Such a situation perpetuates and reinforces childhood dependency, when in fact dependency in this instance is paradoxical, for it is the parent who is mostly dependent on the child for their physical, emotional and constitutional well-being. Thus, children who care are caught in a dependency dilemma. They should – even simply in terms of their development – still be dependants; but they have their own dependants in the form of their sick or disabled parent/s; and yet this does not accord them the status or financial support that we would normally associate with such adult responsibility.

A further significant factor in the uniquely disadvantaged position of child carers is the contradiction inherent in current legislation. This is perhaps surprising, considering the current emphasis on children's rights to advocacy, to equality and to freedom from abuse and neglect (see Alderson 1992; Gulbenkian Foundation Working Group 1993). The Children Act 1989 emphasizes the rights of children, and protection and safety are integral aspects of this (Department of Health 1991). In Section 17, Part III of the Children Act it is stated:

> It shall be the duty of every local authority (a) to safeguard and promote the welfare of children within their area who are in need; and (b) so far as is consistent with that duty, to promote the upbringing of such children by their families, by providing a range and level of services appropriate to those children's needs.

Two particular issues deserve note. First, Section 17(10) of the Act defines a child in need as one who is unlikely to achieve or maintain a 'reasonable standard of health or development' without provision of services by a local authority, or the child's health and development is likely to be 'significantly impaired' without such services. If we apply this criterion to young carers then we cannot deny, and indeed should not be questioning, their status as children in need. However, it is at this point that the divide between definition on the one hand and recognition and provision on the other widens considerably. We might concur that child carers are in need, but this, presently at least, makes little difference to their lives as the provision of services for young carers at a national level is very limited.

Second, the promotion of familial upbringing among young carers is problematic. As we have already discussed, where children are caring for their parents, established notions of parent–child relationships are largely inverted and conventional role models become ambiguous. Although we are not suggesting that children are naturally disadvantaged when a parent is sick or disabled, we are saying that when children have adopted the mantle of responsibility (and accountability) for their parent's welfare, children's lives will inevitably be seriously affected by the impact of such responsibility and role reversal. And yet, at the same time as these roles are confused, children have a right to expect guidance, support and love from their parent/s.

Parents are not being supported in trying to maintain their 'parental responsibilities' in relation to child carers (see Aldridge and Becker 1994a). The current state of policy and service provision is not only failing to serve children who care (and their parents) *appropriately*, it often fails to serve them *at all* (although there are local examples of good practice – see Aldridge and Becker 1994b).

The Community Care guidance (Department of Health 1989; 1990) advocates informal care as an important component of care provision in the community which seems to confuse the protection and safety principles inscribed within the Children Act. Thus, in terms of the legislation, young carers are caught in a caring trap between their position as children and their role as carers.

WAYS FORWARD

Such contradictions in the welfare policies emerging in the 1990s are seen starkly in the twin objectives of the new community care arrangements to control state expenditure (by transferring costs to 'private' individuals and families) and to provide a 'needs-led' service offering 'choice' and 'independence' (Department of Health 1990). The strains of these divergent goals are increasingly seen in the cuts in provision announced by successive local authorities in late 1994 and early 1995 as the annual budget for care became exhausted some months before the end of the financial year (Gilbert 1995). At the time of writing, local authorities are announcing a new round of service reductions and redundancies for 1994/5 as central government grants fail to keep pace with inflation or with the growth in expressed need. Strategies for change, therefore, require not only modifications in current legislation and central government policy, as indicated in the previous section, but also in the level of state resources made available to support informal care generally.

However, while adequate resources may be a necessary condition of improved provision for young carers, it is not a sufficient condition. Even if available, services would not necessarily reach young carers unless the awareness and actions of local authorities, health author-ities and trusts and front line welfare professions also change. For example, local authorities could include the needs of young carers in their community care plans and offer an automatic assessment of the needs of young carers based on their individual requirements.

Awareness-raising strategies in relation to the role young carers play in informal care provision, as well as their rights and needs, are essential both at a national and local level. Such work is already being carried out by Carers National Association Young Carers Project, the Loughborough University Young Carers Research Group, Crossroads and various other local projects and schemes around the country. Now the UN Convention on the Rights of the Child has come into force in the UK, we may also find ways of highlighting the experiences of children who care and emphasizing their rights as children and as carers. Their omission from current legislation has already been highlighted by the Children's Rights Development Unit (CRDU), an independent body set up to monitor the Government's compliance with the Convention (see CRDU 1994: para 5.4.8).

However, when considering the response of legislative and policy developments to the needs of young carers we must be careful to ensure that the consequences of such recognition do not remove child carers from the caring context against their will. Children have said that they want to be both children *and* carers, and to be supported as such (Aldridge and Becker 1993a). For example, decisions about whether tasks are acceptable or unacceptable must lie in negotiation with and within families, in the recognition of both children's and parents' wishes and needs, rather than an imposition of regulations that would prevent children from carrying out certain tasks (even if this were possible). It would be difficult to define and introduce age limits and restrictions on young carers in terms of their caring duties or indeed to set a measure on maturity.

If we cannot decide whether it is acceptable for children to be performing certain caring tasks or caring *per se*, then we must, at least, concur that it is unacceptable for them to continue caring in an environment of disparity and fear. Intervention is needed in order to arrest the disproportionate treatment young carers currently receive from both private and public spheres. Welfare professionals must be aware of their responsibilities to identify, assess and provide services for young carers. It is at the point of contact with families, where children have the potential for providing informal care (such as in those families where long-term illness or disability is present), that professionals should be able to recognize children who might be elected into the caring role and to prevent this by offering appropriate services and by talking with the children and families about what they want. It would thus be possible for appropriately trained and responsive professionals to prevent the unwarranted onset of care provision by children in families.

Supporting and providing for children who are already caring should include: successful negotiation with young carers and their families by welfare professionals; discussion about young carers' needs and the best way to serve and promote them on an individual basis; the removal of threat of familial separation; acknowledgement of their contribution as well as the psychological and physical impact of caring on children (and their families); and recommendations in policy that will emphasize their rights as well as their needs.

From our research it was clear that young carers' needs fall into three distinct areas: someone to talk to; information; and strategic practical help and support. In relation to the first point, it is essential that young carers have access to someone they can talk to in confidence; someone who they can trust *outside* the immediate caring environment but who will understand what it is like to be on the *inside* of caring.

We know the therapeutic value of talking about and sharing problems and anxieties. Sturges (1977: 88) has said: 'Professionals have increasingly recognized how important it can be for children to share their thoughts and feelings about stressful events with their parents or with a therapist.' However, where children are carers they often feel they cannot turn to their parents for such support, as their parents are commonly the source of their anxieties and fears. Furthermore, they do not want to burden their parents with extra worries. Thus, they must have access to independent people who they can turn to as they might turn to a friend, if such friendships were accessible. If young carers have no friends because of the caring commitment, then we should perhaps be helping to create friendships for them, *if that is what they want*. In this respect befriending schemes seem the most appropriate models on which to base this type of support and provision for young carers. One or two such schemes are already being introduced in the UK (see Aldridge and Becker 1994b).

The information needs of young carers are manifest. They urgently need details about support and services (for themselves and for their parents), benefits and welfare advice and, perhaps more significantly, they need medical information. The latter needs to be delivered appropriately and sensitively and, again, taking into account young carers' individual needs and religious, cultural, racial and social backgrounds. The Carers National Association Young Carers Project as well as the Loughborough University Young Carers Research Group have already addressed the information needs of young carers by producing information resource packs for them.

However, such resources need to be reinforced with professional expertise. There are instances where information should be delivered personally in order to deal with the particular circumstances and conditions of young carers and to allay their fears. Thus, GPs and other health professionals should be aware of the experiences and needs of children who care. We have to be particularly cautious with the dissemination of medical information to children when they are carers, for we should not assume that their cognitive understanding is concomitant with their development as carers even though they may have been caring for many years. Many young carers – despite their intimate day to day knowledge of care management practices – are unaware of the nature and implications of the illness/disability they are helping to manage. Some live with fears and concerns about the contagious nature of certain illnesses/disabilities or worries about the prognosis of their parents. Such fears may be amplified by a child's uncertainty and imagination.

In terms of practical support for young carers to help them in their caring routines, an extension of existing services (for example, Community Care Assistant schemes, meals-on-wheels, laundry services, respite care, etc.) would go some way towards relieving some of the stresses inherent in caring. This would require some retraining and awareness-raising among welfare professionals. More significantly, it would require the reassessment of professional attitudes and responses when working with families to recognize, respect and respond to the needs of children who care. The services and support child carers currently receive are scant; it is therefore essential that services are put in place in order to *begin* to benefit these children in the community. The issues generated are wide-ranging and require a reappraisal of who should provide a particular service within a mixed economy of care.

It is imperative that steps are taken to ensure that the young caring experience is not a restricting one, that caring does not seriously constrain young carers' quality of life or their emotional, psycho-social and cognitive development as well as their opportunities to develop and succeed personally and professionally. In the interests of their own health and well-being, young carers have rights as children and as carers and a balance must be struck between their dual roles when planning services and support for them in the community.

REFERENCES

Alderson, P. (1992) 'Rights of children and young people', in Coote, A. (ed.) *The Welfare of Citizens: Developing New Social Rights*, London: Rivers Oram Press.
Aldrige, J. and Becker, S. (1993a) *Children Who Care: Inside the World of Young Carers*, Young Carers Research Group, Loughborough University.

—— (1993b) 'Punishing Children for Caring: The Hidden Cost of Young Carers', *Children and Society* 7 (4): 376–87.

—— (1994a) *My Child, My Carer: The Parents' Perspective*, Young Carers Research Group, Loughborough University.

—— (1994b) *A Friend Indeed: The Case For Befriending Young Carers*, Young Carers Research Group, Loughborough University.

Anthony, E. (1970) 'The Mutative Impact of Serious Mental and Physical Illness in a Parent on Family Life', in Anthony, E. and Koupernik, C. (eds) *The Child In His Family* (Vol. 1), New York: Wiley.

Beard, M. (1975) 'Changing Family Relationships', *Dialysis and Trans-plantation* 4: 36–41.

Biggs, S. (1987) 'Quality of care and the growth of private welfare for old people', *Critical Social Policy* 20: 74–82.

Bilsborrow, S. (1992) *'You Grow Up Fast As Well . . .' Young Carers on Merseyside*, London: Barnardos.

Children's Rights Development Unit (CRDU) (1994) *UK Agenda for Children*, London: CRDU.

Department of Health (1989) *Caring for People: Community Care in the Next Decade and Beyond*, London: HMSO.

—— (1990) *Caring for People: Policy Guidance*, London: HMSO.

—— (1991) *The Children Act 1989 Guidance and Regulations*, London: HMSO.

Gilbert, J. (1995) 'Ways, But No Means', *Nursing Times* 1 February: 13–14.

Gulbenkian Foundation Working Group (1993) *One Scandal Too Many . . . The Case for Comprehensive Protection for Children in all Settings*, Calouste Gulbenkian Foundation: London.

Kossoris, P. (1970) 'Family Therapy', *American Journal of Nursing* 70: 1730–3.

Meredith, H. (1991) 'Developing Support for Young Carers', *The Carer* January: 9.

—— (1992) 'Supporting the Young Carer', *Community Outlook* May: 15–17.

Morris, J. (1993) *Independent Lives: Community Care and Disabled People*, London: Macmillan.

O'Neill, A. (1988) *Young Carers: The Tameside Research*, Tameside: Metropolitan Borough Council.

Office of Population Censuses and Surveys (1992) *General Household Survey of Carers*, London: HMSO.

Page, R. (1988) *Report on the Initial Survey Investigating the Number of Young Carers in Sandwell Secondary Schools*, Sandwell Metropolitan Borough Council.

Patel, N. (1993) 'Healthy Margins: Black Elders' Care – Models, Policies and Prospects', in Ahmad, W.I.U. (ed.) *'Race' and Health in Contemporary Britain*, Milton Keynes: Open University Press.

Sturges, J.S. (1977) 'Talking with Children about Mental Illness in the family', *Health and Social Work of Rehabilitation* 2 (3): 88–109.

Ungerson, C. (1987) *Policy is Personal*, London: Tavistock.

World Health Organization (1982) *Manuals on Child Mental Health and Psychosocial Development*, Geneva: World Health Organization.

Part II

Redistributing resources and control

Chapter 6

Service users acting as agents of change

Clare Evans

INTRODUCTION

As recipients of social care experiencing ill health/impairment, we have traditionally been seen as passive, powerless and dependent on welfare professionals. Excluded from the planning and management of our own care, we have been required to fit into existing patterns of services often inappropriately delivered and varying in quality (Morris 1993). Welfare professionals have tended to make assumptions about our needs based on generalized stereotypes. Moreover, the medical model of disability has been very influential in professional training and thinking and has served to identify the service user as the deviant, rather than stressing society's responsibility not to discriminate (Oliver 1989). Individually we have also not been in a good position to challenge these assumptions, for fear of losing services.

However, through collective action, the disability and psychiatric survivor movement (Oliver 1990; Morris 1991) has challenged and begun to transform this situation. This chapter presents an example of such work, through analysing the achievements of a users' network, of which the author was a founder member, in one locality. The term 'users' is taken to mean those in receipt, on a long-term basis, of provisions for social care, which are essential to a decent existence. The context in which this work has been carried out is the NHS and Community Care Act (1990). This has enshrined service user and carer empowerment in legislation and identified service users as key stakeholders in social care. The emphasis on user empowerment is part of the new consumerist ethos, but as illustrated here, can be used as justification for action to promote users' interests. Such activism does not disregard the fact that fundamental and worsening inequalities in material resources underpin the rationing of provisions for social care (Morris 1993; Whiteley 1995) and the maintenance of control in welfare professionals' hands (Morris 1994). Nevertheless, the account of the development of the Wiltshire Community Care Users' Involvement Network (WCCUIN) which follows, demonstrates that shifts in power relations can be secured which result in services being organized and delivered more in users' interests thereby contributing better to their well-being.

First, the origins of the Network are discussed. Then the significance of the three main sets of strategies employed by the Network in seeking to develop effective user involvement in the management and provision of social care is analysed. The strategies in question are:

• Developing the infrastructure of the Network to reach and involve as many users as possible.
• Proactive approaches to securing effective direct user involvement in policy development and service provision.
• Disseminating what we have learnt.

ORIGINS OF THE NETWORK

In the county of Wiltshire, England, Social Services first attempted to introduce user and carer consultation into the new Community Care planning process in February 1991. Voluntary sector representatives – paid workers apart from two users – and volunteers, met in the countywide Grant Aid Forum of voluntary organizations. The author was asked to chair this conference. However, as a service user, not in touch with other service users, and having difficulty being heard from this perspective at the conference, I found it an isolating experience. Consequently I convened a meeting to discuss user involvement. Four users and their allies attended and their enthusiasm to meet again led to the formation of the Network.

During the next eighteen months I developed contacts for the Network and organized activities from my private house, with small amounts of funding for administrative support and to enable users to meet together. I chaired a Planning Group of ten people, seven of whom were service users from a range of professionally defined care groups and with a wide experience of using services. From the start we sought to maintain the balance between specialist users' groups needing to meet together within the Network, while celebrating the commonality of our disempowerment and the strength and confidence we gained from being one Network. Employing a community development approach, we built up contacts in the Network by encouraging membership from small local self-help groups of users and from individuals, through proactive publicity in voluntary sector newsletters and informal networking (Thornton and Tozer 1994).

By May 1993 we had nearly 300 contacts with individual users and groups of users all over Wiltshire. In recognition of the proactive role we had played in developing user involvement and bringing user perspectives to bear on services, we received £58,000 from Community Care infrastructure funding in a service agreement with Wiltshire Social Services. Funding user-controlled organizations as a means of developing user involvement is identified as good practice by Morris and Lindow (1993). In Wiltshire this grew from an approach to the new Director of Social Services who had arrived in the county at the time the Network was making its initial impact on Social Services. His comments about the value of our work led us to suggest to him that it was an appropriate model of user involvement for the Department, rather than appointing an officer 'in house' to develop a top-down approach.

The purpose of funding in the service agreement was 'to facilitate direct links between users and the Department and to provide a Network of support for service users'. However, from the start we also sought to protect our independence by ensuring that the service agreement was legally binding so that funding could not be withdrawn from the Network as a 'knee jerk' reaction to criticism. We also wrote our own service specification; but, in reality, our belief that such funding would not affect our right to speak out, grew more from the fragile trust that had already developed between users and the Department and joint recognition of the on-going tensions and power imbalances between users and professionals.

One of the results of such understanding developing between the Network and Social Services senior management was the recognition of the enabling role Social Services allies could play when requested to by users (Morris 1994). For example, the problem of viewing empty office properties by a group of users unable to gain physical access to estate agencies was solved by assistance from County Hall staff.

Growing recognition of our work from the local Health Authority, particularly from a few allies involved in collaborative working with the local authority, led, in June 1994, to grant aid of £25,000 for two years. Obtaining more realistic and secure funding for the Network enabled us to take a tenancy on office premises and a meeting room and to employ a Convenor, administrative staff and, later, a Development Worker. We also chose the legal status of a Company Limited by Guarantee and not a charity, for two reasons. First, the Network is based on the principle that it is owned and managed by service users who are paid a small sessional fee for their role in managing the organization and, second, to ensure our campaigning role is not inhibited by rules associated with charity status.

DEVELOPING THE INFRASTRUCTURE OF THE NETWORK

From the start, the right infrastructure of support for users has been vital to developing user involvement on our terms. Having our own organization has been the key to this and secure funding eighteen months after we started made further development possible.

As users, we do not just 'pop up' in response to professional requests for involvement. The users, potential users and ex-users in the Network are often dependent on services on a long-term basis. Many of us have been disempowered and marginalized by society – identified as abnormal and labelled 'disabled'. This affects both our own feelings of self-esteem and the way other members of society react to us. Often too, the bad experiences we have of using services, delivered in a patronizing manner, reinforce these feelings of disempowerment. In order to gain the confidence to give our views, and work with professionals to change services, we need to meet together as users to share experiences and support each other. 'I've never felt safe to say things before' and 'We're not brain-dead after all, are we?' are both comments new recruits to the Network have made after taking part in a meeting with other users. From the start, we have held a regular pattern of meetings on subjects of concern to users, for example, care management, advocacy or transport. The meetings are always chaired by a user and split up into small groups with users chairing each group, demonstrating by this role model the empowerment of users. A few volunteer allies attend as guests of users and if professionals attend to hear our views they do so by invitation. Users' costs in attending are covered, in recognition of the expertise they bring to meetings.

Free membership and a commitment to reach out to and welcome new user members are also important principles we established early on. New members joined us chiefly by self-referral initially or through friends who were members, for workers, whether in the voluntary or statutory sector, appeared not to see the value for users of membership and failed to pass on information. Often small self-help groups were not on the traditional voluntary sector mailing lists and it was necessary to seek out those groups and individual service users by such means as following up newspaper reports. Users experiencing feelings of disempowerment do not become active members by filling in a membership form. Each user is contacted personally, welcomed and the variety of opportunities of involvement explained. Non-users' lack of understanding of the need to reach out to users puts a constant strain on the resources of the staff of our organization who have to facilitate this work as well as negotiating and arranging direct user involvement in service provision.

Now with county-wide membership, we have been able to identify gaps in some areas where no structures exist for groups of users to influence Social Services planning. Active Network members are then able to work with statutory workers to empower users not yet heard. For example, in Western Wiltshire, an initiative to bring together mental health users was started in September 1993. The Network Convenor called a meeting of three mental health users active in the Network, professionals responsible for planning mental health service in Social Services, representatives for the local Health Authority, the local Mental Health NHS Trust and two representatives of voluntary organizations. This group identified the need to bring mental health users together to plan their own ways of influencing services. A series of workshops was subsequently facilitated by mental health users acting as consultants. In preparation for these workshops extensive community development work by a local consultation worker and a social work student on placement with the Network was also carried out. They met users in a variety of settings to encourage them to participate in this initiative. One of their findings was how much the attendance of users in the workshops was affected by the attitude of the staff at the day centres where users went. Staff attitudes varied from failing to agree even to display information publicly for users to learn of this opportunity to speak out, to the other extreme where staff facilitated users' attendance at the workshops by supporting them in making transport arrangements. Such inequalities for users caused by staff attitudes are a recurring problem in our work.

Like every initiative concerned with involving those traditionally excluded from participation in society and having a voice in service provision, this initiative still seems fragile, though the users concerned are committed to continuing to meet together to influence services and a core of users has emerged to take over the running of this group. A joint finance application both to resource continued meetings and development work has also been made by the mental health users co-ordinating the initiative. Meanwhile the pattern of users and professionals working together in equal partnership from the start, to develop the users' voice, has been recognized as a valuable model and is already being used in another part of the county to plan an initiative to bring older service users together.

Service users from ethnic minorities are currently under-represented in the Network and we are anxious not to build structures which perpetuate inequalities and exclude marginalized groups among users. This concern has led us to meet with three local user-led voluntary organizations to develop a proposal with Social Services and the Health Authority to become a national Living Option Partnership site and to employ a worker to enable Asian and African Caribbean disabled people to develop packages of care appropriate to their needs. The outreach work carried out by the development worker has brought the Network into contact with service users in all care groups from the scattered ethnic minority population in Wiltshire which is less than 2 per cent of the total population. This has enabled us to begin to work with a small group of these users to develop appropriate ways for them to get representation.

Underlying all this work to create an organizational infrastructure which supports the empowerment of users is the principle of a bottom up approach – building on the strengths of local user groups and enabling people to have control over their own activities.

DEVELOPING EFFECTIVE USER INVOLVEMENT IN POLICY DEVELOPMENT AND SERVICE PROVISION

Our commitment to be proactive in seeking and creating opportunities for service users to be involved in all aspects of Community Care springs from the belief that a crucial respect in which our right to a quality of life equal to that of other members of society will be achieved, is by users having a direct influence on the services we receive. Only then can changes be made from services which have grown up based on professionals' assumptions of need, to those which offer individuals real choice and control over their lives. This is the perspective of user involvement grounded in full citizenship (Beresford and Croft 1993) and disability as a civil rights issue (Morris 1994). Four initiatives have been central to our making progress on this.

Users taking the lead in policy development

User-led policy development requires considerable time, commitment and energy from users but puts us in a powerful position to influence and shape the future pattern of services.

In 1992, after a Social Services policy document for people with physical disabilities identified obtaining information about need as a priority if delivery of services was to be adequate, the county Joint Commissioning Group of purchasers decided a research project was necessary to identify priorities for new service developments. Users from the Network lobbied for a new pattern of research, with users in each of the three Social Services districts working to identify need and gaps in provision and making recommendations for new services. This work was brought together in a report by a Network member in September 1993. Its principal purchasing recommendations for Joint Finance were the development of a country-wide Information Federation to gather and co-ordinate information and the development of a user-run Information Centre in Salisbury, both under the auspices of the Users' Network. These now represent two out of five user-controlled services managed by the Network and reflect the growing confidence of service users in bidding to take the lead in policy development as a result of their empowerment through the Network.

Power-sharing in resource management: designing Wiltshire Independent Living Fund

There was considerable interest among Network members in the Social Services Committee's decision in March 1993 to involve users in plans to establish a Wiltshire Independent Living Fund (WILF), from money transferred to the Social Services Department within Community Care infrastructure funding. The Network suggested names of members using the Independent Living Fund (providing comprehensive financing for extensive care require- ments) and others with relevant experience, to the officer developing the detailed policy proposals and a working group was set up of eight users, two officers from Social Services and four workers from voluntary organizations. The involvement of users dictated the group's pattern of work, with meetings mid-morning to mid-afternoon with lunch provided, to suit users' transport and care needs. When the detailed policy proposals were complete, users took on responsibility for organizing consultation meetings and the findings of the consultation exercise were incorporated into the final policy proposals.

User influence on the design of policy led to some major differences in the financial criteria for WILF compared with Social Services charging policy. For example, a rule that only the applic- ant's income should be taken into account and not that of the applicant's partner was agreed for WILF. These differing financial criteria caused Social Services management and elected members some concerns on grounds of equity between charging policies. As a result members planned to change the WILF criteria back into line with the department's own criteria when the WILF proposals were brought back to the Social Services Committee for final approval. However, an intensive lobby organized by the Network, of all the members of the Social Services Committee together with a meeting between the users who had designed the proposals and party spokespersons, and a creative suggestion from within the department that the committee consider changing its charging policy to be in line with WILF criteria, led to a unanimous decision by all Social Services Committee members to support the users' proposals! The misunderstandings that arose between the Network and Social Services senior management during this work were at times frus- trating and painful, but mutual efforts to unravel these and a successful resolution of the impasse, led to increased trust between the organizations.

Now Wiltshire Independent Living Fund is established independ- ently in the community and operates with a grants panel of disabled people making decisions about applications on a monthly basis. In 1995/6 the funding allocated to be used by individuals to enable them to live independently in the community amounts to nearly £1 million. Neither the professionals nor users involved would have believed at the start of their work in designing the WILF, the degree to which the scheme would be established under user control. However, the openness with which both service users and Social Services staff were prepared to work, led to the removal of barriers to participation and power-sharing unimaginable a year earlier. The appropriateness of users having control over a scheme which will enable disabled people to have, to a greater extent, the quality of life to which they are entitled seems correct!

Developing user-controlled services

In addition to the two information projects mentioned earlier, three further proposals for projects to be developed within the Network have obtained funding. A support service for people starting to use the Wiltshire Independent Living Fund is designed to draw on the experience of people already using cash payments to live independently in the community. A further project provides people from ethnic minority communities with appropriate support to gain access to WILF. A fifth project utilizes the experience of mental health service users to develop a Patients' Council in a psychiatric hospital. All the projects are based in service delivery areas in which users have expertise within their life experience such as advocacy and independent living. Our belief that service users can develop alternative, more sensitive ways of delivering services will be systematically measured over the next three years. The importance of developing appropriate and user-led methods of evaluation is now being addressed.

User input to care management procedures

The philosophy of care management – assessment of needs with the user and the development of a care plan to meet those needs – should in theory give us the opportunity of gaining independence from professional assumptions about our requirements. The challenge of Wiltshire Social Services Department in 1993 was to produce procedures reflecting this philosophy. Over the two-year period since professionals first began designing the procedures, the increased influence and power of the Network has enabled us to work with them to influence this design and the attitudes of care managers.

The first new referral and assessment forms were designed without users contributing and were brought to a Network meeting at our request, for consultation. The anger at their inappropriateness was considerable and following that, a much closer working relationship was developed with the Network. A series of workshops was organized for users to contribute to key stages of the process – designing the care plan form, revising the referral and assessment forms, discussing the Review process and developing a document setting out users' principles for care management. These workshops were funded initially by the Social Services Department and after April 1993, when our funding was agreed, from within our own budget, to give us more control over the nature of our involvement. In addition to costs for attending the workshops, users were paid an hourly rate for the expertise they brought to them.

No procedures, however well designed, can be developed appropriately unless the attitude of the staff responsible also reflects what should be the underlying philosophy. To brief Social Services and Health professionals who were to become care managers from April 1993, a programme of training days on assessment and care planning had been planned by the Social Services Department. Following two users' participation in a pilot training day, the Network prepared a short paper proposing user participation in all the forthcoming training days. The paper laid down the good practice users would expect in order to participate – such as at least two users attending each day, accessible venues, the opportunity for preparatory learning and debriefing, users' costs reimbursed and an hourly fee to value the expertise they brought. The proposal with its cost implications was agreed by the Director of Social Services and immediately we began to draw up a list of those users who were interested in participating in such training. Over fifty users participated in these training days over an eighteen-month period and the subsequent pattern of staff training has continued to adopt this model of user participation.

The Wiltshire model of user involvement in training – that of users as equal participants on training days designed round group work to which they can contribute user expertise – is an effective way of involving a range of users with a variety of perspectives. It prevents accusations of only the most articulate users being involved. This is often professionals' defence against recognizing the value of users in training. It means we have a pool of users immediately available to participate and enables users to learn with professionals about assessment and care planning in Community Care. It has been effective in breaking down stereotyped views. Frequently users perceive that professionals' attitudes change during a training day, as the users' expertise is recognized. Feedback from Trainers and Care Managers indicates that they have also recognized this change in their perception of users.

As management of Community Care is devolved within Social Services and as users develop more links with the Health Authority, changing patterns of user involvement in review procedures are emerging. In addition to involvement at county level, such as users participating in the monthly meeting of the newly formed Social Services Performance Quality Unit, we are supporting users' participation in local inter-professional community care implementation groups and inter-agency Service Review groups such as those concerning the Occupational Therapy service. For all the users involved in such activities, the Network is there to support them financially, to enable them to network with other users to learn from their experience and to provide them with independent information and support between meetings.

DISSEMINATING WHAT WE HAVE LEARNT

At a time when there is considerable commitment to the concept of user involvement but some difficulty in 'getting started', we have felt it important that as users we ourselves contribute to developing good practice by disseminating the lessons we have learnt from our experience within the Network.

As interest in the Network has grown we receive several enquiries a week about our work from statutory and voluntary sector personnel and organizations of service users. We send out packs about our work to enquirers, we run bi-monthly seminars on our work and we accept invitations to speak at conferences in other local authorities. The additional income generated by our charges for these services provides a useful source of independent funding which we can use for campaigning activity, such as support for the introduction in Britain of comprehensive anti-discriminatory legislation for disabled people. Such campaigning we see not as an extra, but as part of our core work to bring about more equal participation, not only in Community Care but in society in general.

To reach the social workers of tomorrow – to ensure they learn good practice concerning user empowerment in their initial training – is a valuable way of improving services and decreasing inequalities in the future. We now have links with social work qualifying courses at Bristol University, Bath University, Bournemouth University and

Trowbridge College. There are particularly strong links with Bristol University where eight Network members have given lectures and a student has been on placement with the Network. The senior lecturer with whom we negotiate our involvement wrote, 'The direct testimony of users and their teaching role has a significant effect on the opportunities for students to learn about users' views.'

Funding from the Central Council for Education and Training of Social Work has also enabled us to develop a regional network of users acting as trainers and to become an accredited provider of training. Certainly, service users within the Network echo others who have contributed to changing the culture of training in stressing the importance of user involvement (Beresford 1994).

CONCLUSIONS

The key to the effectiveness of Wiltshire Community Care User Involvement Network in bringing about changes which reduce inequalities in Health and Social Services provision through user involvement in Community Care, lies in the Network's ability to raise the self-esteem of people whom society has marginalized. The confidence gained through consciousness-raising, by linking personal distress and disability to a shared recognition of our own oppression, has enabled us to take advantage of the undefined concepts of user involvement and user empowerment enshrined in the Community Care legislation and to challenge the traditional service recipient's role.

The receptiveness and understanding we have found among service allies within the Social Services Department and more recently in the Health Authority concerning our specific role and the value of collective user involvement, have enabled us to secure funding with which to establish a broad base of user participation. This has begun to change the attitude and culture of local welfare agencies towards a more equal relationship with service users.

The energy and expertise of service users supported by our own organization, combined with the commitment of senior welfare professionals to use their personal power to enable us to gain a position of power and influence, has given us a vision of user-controlled services characterized by users' choice and control and the recognition of users as major stake-holders. The future will show whether users' energy and expertise, together with allies' commitment, is strong enough to resist the constraints of rationing, lack of resources and society's expectations of welfare agencies as agents of social control, to bring about long-term changes in inequalities in service provision.

REFERENCES

Beresford, P. (1994) *Changing the Culture*, London: Central Council for Education and Training in Social Work.

Beresford, P. and Croft, S. (1993) *Citizen Involvement – A Practical Guide For Change*, Birmingham/Basingstoke: BASW/Macmillan.

Morris, J. (1991) *Pride Against Prejudice*, London: The Women's Press.

—— (1993) *Community Care or Independent Living?* York: Joseph Rowntree Foundation.

—— (1994) *The Shape of Things to Come? User-led Social Services*, London: National Institute of Social Work.

Morris, J. and Lindow, V. (1993) *User Participation in Community Care Services*, London: Community Care Support Force, Department of Health.

Oliver, M. (1989) 'Disability and dependency: a creation of industrial societies?' in Barton, L. (ed.) *Disability and Dependency*, London: The Falmer Press.

—— (1990) *The Policies of Disablement*, London: Macmillan.

Thornton, P. and Tozer, R. (1994) *Involving Older People in Planning and Evaluating Community Care*, York: Social Policy Research Unit, York University.

Whiteley, P. (1995) 'Department of Health acknowledges crisis', *Community Care* 6–11 January: 1.

Chapter 7

Localities and inequalities
Locality management in the inner-city

Rosie Weaver

INTRODUCTION

The organization and delivery of health care in Britain has been undergoing the most fundamental and rapid changes since the inception of the National Health Service (NHS). Through the introduction of market principles into the management and control of health care, it is proposed that 'consumers' will be able to exercise greater choice and enjoy more effective, efficient and responsive provision. The overt aims of the reformed NHS are to target services at locally identified needs within the resources available, to assess and respond to individual need and to offer treatment and care in partnership with users, their families and carers through inter-agency collaboration in order to provide high quality services (Department of Health 1989a, 1989b, 1989c, 1991, NHS Management Executive 1993).

However, Government proposals for the 'New NHS' are likely to be undermined by two key factors: first, because they pay little attention to the significance of social inequalities or health inequalities for *The Health of the Nation* (Department of Health 1992), in the face of the growing evidence of the impact of intense local pockets of deprivation (Phillimore *et al.* 1994; Davey Smith and Morris 1994) and, second, because the introduction of GP fundholding and NHS Trusts has multiplied the difficulties involved in securing a co-ordinated local response to identified health needs.

Health service managers are in the front line of these contradictions between the rhetoric and the reality of the NHS and may, at the local level, bring a perspective which is at odds with the direction proposed by Government and the NHS Executive. This chapter considers the contribution health service managers might make to combating health inequalities by analysing the author's experience as a 'locality manager'. It describes the findings of a detailed social and health profile of the area for which the author was responsible and evaluates a series of projects designed to counteract the impact of inequalities on the health of the local population. Finally, it discusses the formidable obstacles to improving the health of the local population which were presented by a rapid succession of destructive reorganizations.

WHAT IS LOCALITY MANAGEMENT?

The organization of community primary care services on a 'patch' or 'locality' basis was identified in the Cumberlege Report (Department of Health 1986) as a model of identifying and responding to local needs in a flexible way, reflecting inequalities in health status between areas. Primary Health Care has been defined as 'the developing range of NHS services . . . which are provided in the home, the surgery and the community by family health services (the family doctors, nurse practitioners, practice nurses, dentists, retail pharmacists and optometrists) and the community health services (community nurses, midwives, health visitors and other professions allied to medicine)' (North East Thames Regional Health Authority 1991).

This example of 'Locality Management' developed from a twelve-month pilot project between the Family Health Service Authority (FHSA) and the South Birmingham Health Authority (SBHA) Community Unit born of the recognition that both organizations needed to work together to provide primary health care services. Initially, the Locality Management Team (LMT) comprised three Primary Health Care Managers, a Practice Nurse Adviser, a GP Adviser, a Public Health Consultant and a Business Support Manager led by a 'Locality Manager' and answerable to the Unit General Manager. Communication channels between GPs, practice nurses and community staff were strengthened and local conflicts between the FHSA and the SBHA were able to be resolved using the advice of team members. The LMT had no formal links to the Local Authority, but invited representatives of Local Authority services (and representatives of professional and voluntary groups) to discuss specific issues.

The Locality Manager was faced, from the outset, with at least three key strategic problems. First, it is not just NHS provision which can influence the health of a local population. As a recent report on primary care in Birmingham states, 'the mainstream programmes of the City Council's service provision such as urban regeneration, housing improvement, environmental, health and social services have a huge impact' (Bosanquet 1993: 30). Second, effective co-ordination of the services provided by local councils, health services and voluntary and private bodies has long been difficult to realize in practice. Morever, third, improved co-ordination may have a contribution to make to improving the health of a local population but this is unlikely to be a sufficient reponse when pursued in isolation from or in opposition to national policy. Locality managers face the question of what can be achieved to combat the effects of structural inequalities *on* a relatively small local area and the effects of inequalities between people *within* such an area, when national, or even regional, economic and social policies are beyond their control.

SPARKBROOK LOCALITY PROFILE

One of the key elements in Locality Management is that it provides the structure to develop an in-depth profile of the constituency. Such a profile is designed to help identify key factors influencing the health of the population and smaller areas and groups facing particular obstacles to securing good health, as a basis for planned intervention. Sparkbrook Constituency had a total population of 75, 500 in 1991 (Office of Population Censuses and Surveys 1993). Of these residents, 9.4 per cent were under five, and over 27 per cent were under fifteen. Just under one in twenty were seventy-five or over. The locality is made up of three electoral wards containing roughly similar numbers of people: Sparkbrook, Sparkhill and Fox Hollies.

Using local knowledge, networking with statutory and voluntary agencies and collating data used by them together with census data, an analysis of the profile of Sparkbrook was developed by the Locality Management Team (LMT). The data collected clearly identified, on a number of measures, high levels of relative disadvantage in the constituency compared to the wider population and differences between the three wards. For example, in terms of two composite indices of deprivation, the Jarman Score[1] and the Townsend Score[2], Sparkbrook ward recorded the highest level of deprivation in South Birmingham (Jarman 1983, 1984; Townsend 1987).

Table 7.1 Jarman and Townsend Scores in the Sparkbrook constituency by ward

	Jarman Score	Townsend Score
Fox Hollies	34	5.87
Sparkbrook	50	12.10
Sparkhill	37	8.75

Such composite scores reflect, but also hide, detailed evidence of the material obstacles to health faced by residents in Sparkbrook. These details were explored in other information collected by the LMT, for example, in terms of housing, unemployment levels and poverty.

Housing

With variations, the 1991 census indicates that the overall standard of the housing stock was poor, especially in the Sparkhill and Sparkbrook wards. In terms of overcrowding, lack of amenities, house ownership and homelessness, people living in the constituency faced high levels of difficulty. Overcrowding (defined as over one person per room) in Sparkbrook ward is the highest in the City of Birmingham while all three wards have above average levels.

Table 7.2 Households with over one person per room by ward (per cent)

Fox Hollies	4.2
Sparkbrook	13.5
Sparkhill	10.4
City Average	4.0

Source OPCS Census of Population 1991

Absent or difficult-to-use sanitation, also has an adverse impact on health. Table 7.3 shows that the Sparkhill ward, especially, has a high percentage of houses without basic amenities. Despite the establishment of Housing Action Areas and General Improvement Areas, approximately three-quarters of all properties were in need of improvement.

Of the permanent households in the constituency 50.5 per cent were owner-occupied, 10.8 per cent privately rented, 10.4 per cent rented from Housing Associations and 27.3 per cent rented from the local authority. In the Sparkbrook Ward only 35 per cent of private

Table 7.3 Households lacking bath/shower and/or inside wc by ward (per cent)

Fox Hollies	1.4
Sparkhill	4.6
Sparkbrook	1.8
City Average	1.5

Source OPCS Census of Population 1991

households were owner occupied. House prices in the area were high, even for deteriorating properties, compared with other inner-city locations. Buying a house was, therefore, beyond the means of people on low incomes. Sparkhill and Sparkbrook were popular areas for Asian families because of family and religious ties and the availability of a range of familiar goods and services.

The pressure on housing was further exemplified in the homelessness statistics for the area measured during the period January–June 1991. With 37.4 priority-need homeless cases per 1,000 households, Sparkbrook ward had the second highest concentration of homeless cases in Birmingham.

Unemployment

Table 7.4 shows that there was a high level of unemployment in the Sparkhill and Sparkbrook wards. Sparkbrook has the highest level of any ward in Birmingham and three times the European Community average.

Table 7.4 Unemployed by ward (per cent)

Fox Hollies	14.0
Sparkbrook	32.6
Sparkhill	22.5
City Average	14.3

Source OPCS Census of Population 1991

Poverty

The proportion of households with no car is a good indicator of disposable income as well as indicating difficulties accessing services. Table 7.5 shows the differences between wards and the comparison with the city as a whole.

Table 7.5 Households with no car by ward (per cent)

Fox Hollies	49.6
Sparkhill	50.7
Sparkbrook	68.7
City Average	45.1

Source: OPCS Census of Population 1991

Another measure of low income is the level of eligibility for free school meals. In the Sparkbrook ward 53 per cent of children were eligible, the third highest proportion in the city.

Ethnic minority status

Ethnic minority group residents were more likely to be found in the wards with high levels of deprivation (Table 7.6) where, indeed, they were not in the minority! To direct resources into these wards was likely to coincidentally result in those resources being directed at members of minority ethnic groups. Other data made it clear that, for a substantial minority of these residents, communication in English was difficult.

Table 7.6 Ethnic minority status by ward (per cent)

	White	African Caribbean/ African	Asian	Other
Fox Hollies	86	4	10	1
Sparkhill	38	7	53	3
Sparkbrook	33	13	48	6
City Average	78	6	14	2

Source: OPCS Census of Population 1991

Key health indicators

It is not surprising that the Locality Management Team found that the high levels of deprivation were reflected in a high level of mortality. Statistics produced by South Birmingham Health Authority for the period 1986–9 showed that Sparkhill and Sparkbrook had the highest rates of infant deaths of all South Birmingham wards (17.4 and 15.6 per 1,000 live births, respectively) and Sparkhill had the largest number of stillbirths (Healthy Birmingham 2000 1993).

Statistics on death in the first year of life are amongst the most sensitive indicators of the health of a population (Blackburn 1991).

Amongst adults, Sparkbrook had the highest rates of death from heart disease, lung cancer and accidents within the South Birmingham Health Authority area. For the period 1986–91, Sparkbrook ward had the highest Standardized Mortality Ratio in Birmingham for all causes of death in the age group 25–74 (men: 183; women: 159). Birmingham as a whole was above the national average.

PROJECTS TO COMBAT SOCIAL AND HEALTH INEQUALITIES

This analysis of the area, together with evidence drawn from the experience of front line staff and from other research about health prevention and promotion led to the identification by the Locality Management Team of priorities for improving provision, for example, to respond to the diversity of population groups in the area. In turn, these resulted in a series of developments led by the Locality Manager or the Primary Care Managers on the LMT. These either used new sources of funding, such as Inner-city Partnership money, or involved the reorganization of existing services. The five projects discussed here, examples of a larger number of actions taken, illustrate some of the key priorities of the LMT, namely, to:

- increase access to health information;
- improve access to health services; and
- empower service users to influence and develop services to meet their health needs.

Access through interpreters

The locality profile had identified that, for a large proportion of the population, English was not a first language. The availability of interpreters is vital if users of NHS health services who are non-English speaking and, therefore, face communication difficulties with health professionals are to be offered equality of access. The practice of using family members to interpret on the individual's behalf also raises other concerns including lack of confidentiality. From the LMT's point of view, if local health initiatives were to be effective, they needed to reach this substantial proportion of the population.

In Sparkbrook, the demand for interpreters for work in people's homes, at clinics and in health promotion activities via groups and exhibitions, far exceeded supply. Moreover, the existing staffing did not cover the range of languages needed. When the LMT monitored the interpreting service over a six-month period it was found that there were peaks and troughs of demand for different languages, with the effect that at times some interpreters were under-utilized. It was evident that a reorganization of interpreting services was needed so that the limited resources could be used more effectively for the benefit of service users.

The key outcome of this review was to establish the need for continuing interpreter posts covering a number of 'core' languages – Punjabi, Hindi, Bengali and Urdu – while a 'bank' system was developed to cover other languages. Sessional interpreting posts were advertised in the local press with a good response rate. It was recognized that a system of employing 'bank' staff could be viewed as discriminatory as these staff could not enjoy the conditions of service of permanent staff members. A comprehensive in-house certificated training programme was developed for both permanent and bank interpreters, as well as training for community nursing staff in how to work alongside interpreters and to use this resource effectively.

This reorganization has helped the locality to move away from *ad hoc* usage of interpreting staff to a more co-ordinated and comprehensive approach to meeting the needs of people whose first language is not English. Evidence of the impact of this project is found in the increasing demand for interpreters from professionals working in the area, which has led to an increase in the range of languages offered, and in the purchasing of the interpreter service by the FHSA for use by GPs.

Improving access via the Immunization and Cervical Cytology Project

Another issue of equal access was addressed through the Immunization and Cervical Cytology Project. The decision to focus attention on immunization and cervical cytology screening services in Sparkbrook, was based on evidence from General Practices of low uptake in an area containing a high number of children under fifteen as well as the attention paid to these issues in *The Health of the Nation* (Department of Health 1992). Inner-city Partnership funding was secured for a three-year joint project with the Family Health Service Authority and the District Health Authority to improve uptake of these services within the wards of Sparkhill and Sparkbrook amongst women from Black and minority ethnic groups. Particular areas and General Practices were targeted where uptake was low.

The project focused on raising public awareness of these two important health issues by the following means:

• establishing a network of contacts and identifying key people and organizations within the locality with the potential to influence health;
• obtaining access to as many groups as possible within the area and establishing health education programmes;
• planning specific health education programmes in liaison with local schools;
• visiting every General Practice which has low uptake, offering fact sheets, videos, posters and leaflets in a range of languages;
• providing information directly to women in these practices' waiting rooms; and
• discussing ways of improving uptakes and removing barriers to access with Primary Health Care teams and with women themselves;

How successful was the project in terms of activity and outcomes? Within two years, the project team of a Health Visitor, a Link worker and an Interpreter visited 168 groups and were involved in forty-eight community exhibitions at Women's Day events, cultural centre celebrations, parents' evenings, leisure centres and neighbourhood offices, to name but a few. Over 4,100 people were contacted through these venues. General Practitioners, educational and religious organizations welcomed the project team and a committed participatory approach was adopted. New resources have been developed: for example, a community video 'Important Appointments' has been dubbed in Urdu/Bengali, leaflets have been printed in Arabic on immunization and cervical cytology and audio tapes produced on cervical screening for travelling families.

Outcomes have been evaluated by reviewing uptake data and through two surveys. The numbers of people attending health clinics and the numbers of children who completed their 'primaries', the course of three sets of combined immunization against Polio, Pertussis, Diphtheria and Tetanus, have increased every year since 1991. More women are receiving cervical smear tests and more children are being immunized. However, the figures collected by the FHSA show that the uptake of the pre-school booster remains low.

A survey of women's knowledge before contact with the project team found that 70 to 80 per cent of women had some knowledge of cervical smears. Knowledge about the suggested frequency for testing and how to obtain and understand results was more limited. There was also evidence to suggest that the older women were less likely to present for regular smear tests.

The second survey to check the impact of the project asked women how they felt about the project and the information they had received. Eighty per cent of women reported that the information was useful and they felt better informed, 50 per cent said they would go for a smear on a regular basis, and 60 per cent said they would encourage other women to attend for smear tests. Nearly 99 per cent of the women wanted more information on other health issues, for example, breast cancer, diabetes and childhood asthma.

The project has confirmed the desire amongst women for more information about immunization and cervical screening and that there are gaps in public knowledge. Statistical returns (not available for publication) showed that the methods adopted resulted in increased take-up of the targeted services. Future health education sessions have been planned to meet the information needs identified by women who were in contact with the Project Team.

Increasing access through user involvement and advocacy

This approach to evaluating the immunization and cervical screening project by asking users' opinions was part of a wider strategy to 'empower' service users through providing information, consultation, participation and giving users a measure of control over the services they receive. The LMT sought to find ways in which the requirement of purchasers of services (GP Fundholders and District Health Authorities) to demonstrate that they were responding to local needs, would be used to establish mechanisms for involving local residents in saying what they felt about existing services and what they wanted for the future.

For example, users' views were sought by questionnaires and interviews about local community nursing services. Some opinions were relatively easily acted on, for example, the desire for access to interpreters when attending a clinic or when a district nurse or health visitor called, as discussed earlier. However, translating user views into decisions is clearly a complex issue where there are many diverse groups of users with different expectations and perceptions of health needs, which can conflict with purchasers' and providers' views. One example concerned a choice about the best time of day for a 'well baby' clinic. Some users wanted the clinic to run in the evening and at weekends, while others preferred clinic sessions in the morning. Evening and weekend working is more expensive both in staffing and in the costs associated with opening health centres and GP surgeries. Hence cost effectiveness became a critical issue in reaching a decision. Purchasing decisions are supposed to be based on well founded information about health concerns of the local population, but where tensions exist between managing health costs and local responsiveness, it is the purchasers who make final choices.

The LMT have supported a number of local advocacy initiatives. Advocacy is designed to redress inequalities in power within a locality by helping groups and individuals challenge assumptions, define and fight for their rights, influence decisions and, thereby, secure services that better meet their requirements. Advocacy projects have been developed on a 'client group' basis, for example, with people with a learning disability and with older people with mental health problems and on a 'social group' basis, for example, with the Yemeni community.

The Yemeni Health Advocacy Project is still in its infancy. It was identified that all services had been poor at responding to the particular health needs of this small community. Arabic-speaking interpreters, health education information and information on GP, Hospital and Health Centre services in Arabic had been non-existent. A Steering Group was set up with representatives from the Yemeni community, Birmingham City Council Race Relations Unit, the FHSA and the LMT, together with a local GP and a health visitor, to guide the work undertaken by a project worker. Her role was to increase the health information provided to the Yemeni community by networking with groups of women, supporting them in attending health appointments and accessing services and identifying unmet health needs.

The project worker worked alongside health professionals in setting up new local groups and accessing those already in existence, for example, English and sewing classes. The women requested more information on a variety of health issues including immunization, womens' health and understanding the hospital and health clinic appointments systems. Joint work was done with the local Islamic

Resource Centre to translate health education leaflets into Arabic as well as information about where the local health centres and GPs were located. It is also planned to make audio tapes in Arabic.

It is envisaged that the project will provide a source of feedback on the quality and quantity of services the Yemeni community presently receive and a means of influencing future planning of services to meet their specific needs. It will also help members of the community to access present services more easily.

Ideally, the funding of such advocacy projects should be independent of service providers and not time limited, but experience nationally shows that this is at best very difficult to secure. Two of the advocacy projects in Sparkbrook have time-limited funding, one from Joint Finance arrangements and the other from Inner-city Partnership funds.

Increasing access by reorganizing local services

In addition to attempts to secure improved access to existing services, the LMT was concerned to ensure that such services were best organized to meet need. Community nursing services had been delivered on a geographical basis which meant that several community staff liaised with several GPs. In order to develop stronger primary health care teams as a basis for identifying and addressing health care needs in the practice, Sparkbrook community nursing services were reorganized and aligned to the GP practices in Sparkbrook. Each GP practice in Sparkbrook now had a named health visitor and a named district nurse teamleader for that surgery. Patients as well as the practice staff knew who to access and how, much more easily. Examples of the benefits included:

- easier access for parents to health visitors by the development of baby clinics in surgeries and some health visitors being practice-based;
- practice-specific health promotion activities such as a weaning clinic; and
- joint work between community staff and practice nurses resulting in developments such as asthma clinics and leg ulcer clinics.

However, the dispersal of GP practice populations through a number of wards meant that basing services on practices could conflict with attempts to co-ordinate services within local geographical communities.

CURRENT AND FUTURE HEALTH STRATEGIES

Despite these and other initiatives, attempts to establish effective Locality Management have been undermined by the continuing pace of change in the organization of the NHS and by the introduction of economic incentives to induce different elements of the Service to act competitively rather than co-operatively. Locality Management, which only began in Sparkbrook in April 1992, had been subject to three major organizational changes by April 1995.

When the local services obtained Trust status in 1994, it was recognized that there was an inherent conflict of interest between the new Community Health Trust as provider of services and both the Birmingham Family Health Service Authority (FHSA) and the District Health Authority as purchasers of services. GP fundholders were to be rewarded for improved primary health care delivery only to their own patients, with no incentive to think in terms of the locality, while there was no guarantee that Fundholders would continue to purchase services from the local provider Trust. Where community services were purchased from outside the immediate area, patients of that practice were ineligible for any of the community services provided by the local Trust such as advice from a clinic nearer to where they live. Consequently, joint management arrangements became untenable and inter-agency co-operation to improve services within a locality was significantly threatened.

In Sparkbrook, the basic approach of Locality Management was continued within the new Southern Birmingham Community Trust. Each locality was then solely managed by Locality Managers responsible for ensuring that existing contracts were met and that business plans of the Division were rooted in local health needs information. They directly managed all district nurses, health visitors and school nurses and administrative staff. Services managed outside the Locality Division were co-ordinated by them.

Contemporaneously, the strategy document 'Birmingham 1995: A Strategy for Primary Care' commissioned by the FHSA and published in 1993, proposed a Constituency Action Programme approach which again identified small geographical areas as the unit for managing and planning primary care. Constituency Action Teams (CAT) were set up in 1993, in each of the twelve parliamentary constituencies in Birmingham, with representatives from the various services provided by the Local Authority (Housing, Leisure and Recreation, Social Services, Environmental Services, Architecture and Planning, and Education), the Community Health Council (who represented users), the Mental Health Trust, the Community Trust, the District Health Authority, the FHSA and a GP. Each CAT was charged with identifying and prioritizing the primary health care needs of the local population in order to bid for money allocated by the Regional Health Authority for primary health care. One of the major benefits of CATs was that planning health care on a local basis was done across agency boundaries.

This approach is still in its infancy and debate abounds as to whether it will reach adulthood. To date, the bids are being scrutinized by relevant purchasing teams in Birmingham and the FHSA. Whether there is a resource allocation based on links between deprivation and identified health needs is still an unanswered question. For local managers and practitioners in Sparkbrook, this allocation would seem a perfect opportunity to address some of the inequalities in health.

Meanwhile another report, 'Spotlight on Primary Care', commissioned by the Regional Health Authority (West Midlands Health 1994), proposed an alternative vision for primary care. It suggested a new model of Primary Care Units which would be responsible for providing (and where necessary purchasing) primary care and for purchasing secondary care for a defined registered population, generally one or more GP practice lists. The Unit would consist of a team of health care professionals – GPs, dentists, practice nurses, community nurses, health visitors and midwives, pharmacists, opticians, social workers, paramedical staff. This could mean the demise of the Community Trust as it exists at present, with Locality Management becoming a redundant concept. The place of inter-agency working via the CAT teams and of user involvement is uncertain.

Over the same period as these changes, successive 'restructuring' by the FHSA and the Trust have meant, first, the deletion of the Practice Nurse Adviser post on the LMT, second, the redundancy of the Business Support Manager and, third, the loss of six management posts within the 'Localities Division' of the Trust.

CONCLUSION

Locality Management has offered a basis for Health Service managers to work to meet the health needs of a local population. Health care management based on a limited geographical area has a number of key advantages:

- detailed knowledge of local areas and communities and closer working relationships with colleagues in other agencies operating in the same area, leading to easier identification of local health issues and better access for local people both to named professionals directly providing services and also to known managers and planners of services, because they are based within the area;
- locality-based inter-agency strategies can be more effective than those acting at a local council to health authority level because they work through middle managers with direct, operational responsibility for service provision and are at a scale which allows for detailed knowledge of – and response to – the population needs;
- service users, whose involvement is vital to the development of effective and appropriate services, can identify with services which are provided locally from centres which they can access directly in places they are used to frequent; and
- the geographical basis for service planning and delivery provided a focus for identifying health concerns linked to economic and social inequalities, involving local people in identifying health concerns linked to economic and social inequalities, involving local people in identifying needs and service shortfalls and creating a relevant, co-ordinated inter-agency response.

In Sparkbrook, a series of projects aimed at improving access to and the quality of service provision by engaging with service users and tackling the structural inequalities which affect health, began to demonstrate the possible benefits of the approach. However, some formidable obstacles emerged. First, the introduction of further changes in the organizational structures and the management ideology of the NHS introduced sets of competing and conflicting interests which threaten to bring Locality Management to an end and undermine the work undertaken. Both the rate of change and the underlying ideology behind the changes are at odds with the development of responsive, appropriate, user-led services. The image suggested is the professionally managed supermarket rather than the workers' co-operative. The crucial difference is to whom the management is accountable.

Second, the increasing number of bodies involved in planning for or providing National Health Services to a particular population (Health Authorities, Hospital and Community Trusts, budget-holding and non-budget-holding GPs and FHAs) created additional problems for the development of a co-ordinated strategy to combat local health inequalities, especially as these bodies have a variety of other, sometimes conflicting interests.

Third, these problems were compounded by the differences in political control and management and professional ideologies between the locally elected city council and the centrally appointed health authorities. Sparkbrook is now the proposed European URBAN pilot project in the City of Birmingham, part of a greater Area Regneration Initiative that includes Sparkbrook, Sparkhill and neighbouring Tyseley. The development of the URBAN proposals have involved a high level of public participation and empowerment and has brought together organizations, businesses, individuals and community groups in addressing issues of community regeneration intended to provide an increased range of training opportunities and employment prospects. It is significant that the LMT was not invited to be directly involved in these Local Authority-led plans for the economic regeneration of the area which would also have a significant effect on the health of the people of Sparkbrook by addressing underlying disadvantage.

As in work reported in other chapters, the Locality Management approach has demonstrated the significance of user involvement as a springboard for equalizing access to and experience of health care as a contribution to equalizing health chances. It demonstrates the possibilities offered by local action but reveals the capacity for wider national political and economic policies to undermine and ultimately terminate such developments.

NOTES

1 The Jarman Score is a composite indicator based on census data which indicates relative scores of deprivation. It is based on:

- The percentage of lone parents;
- The percentage aged under five;
- The percentage of single parent households;
- The percentage of people in social class V;
- The percentage unemployed;
- The percentage in crowded households (more than one per room);
- The percentage of people who have moved in the last year; and
- The percentage of people in non-White ethnic groups.

(Jarman 1983, 1984)

2 The Townsend Score is an alternative measure of social deprivation. The score is an unweighted average of four census variables, indexed to England. The variables are:

- The percentage of households not owner-occupied;
- The percentage of households without a car;
- The percentage of households with more than one person per room;
- The percentage unemployed.

(Townsend 1987)

REFERENCES

Blackburn, C. (1991) *Poverty and Health: Working with Families*, Milton Keynes: Open University Press.

Bosanquet, N. (1993) *Primary Care in Birmingham: A Strategy for Primary Care*, Birmingham: Birmingham City Council.

Davey Smith, G. and Morris, J. (1994) 'Increasing Inequalities in the Health of the Nation', *British Medical Journal* 309: 1453–4.

Department of Health (1986) *Neighbourhood Nursing: A Focus for Care*, London: HMSO.

—— (1989a) *Working for Patients*, London: HMSO.

—— (1989b) *Caring for People*, London: HMSO.

—— (1989c) *General Practice in the New NHS. A New Contract*, London: HMSO.

—— (1991) *The Patient's Charter: Raising the Standard*, London: HMSO.

—— (1992) *The Health of the Nation: A Strategy for Health in England*, London: HMSO.

Healthy Birmingham 2000 (1993) 'Health Inequalities in Birmingham', Report to the Birmingham Joint Consultative Health Committee, Birmingham: Healthy Birmingham 2000.

Jarman, B. (1983) 'Identification of underprivileged areas', *British Medical Journal* 286: 1705–9.

—— (1984) 'Underprivileged areas: validation and distribution of scores', *British Medical Journal* 289: 1587–92.

NHS Management Executive (1993) *A Vision for the Future: The Nursing, Midwifery and Health Visiting Contribution to Health and Health Care*, London: Department of Health.

North East Thames Regional Health Authority (1991) *Primary Care in the 90s – A Strategic Statement*, London: North East Thames Regional Health Authority.

Office of Population Censuses and Surveys (1993) *Decennial Census 1991*, London: HMSO.

Phillimore, P., Beattie, A. and Townsend, P. (1994) 'Widening inequality of health in northern England 1981–91', *British Medical Journal* 308: 1125–32.

Townsend, P. (1987) 'Deprivation', *Journal of Social Policy* 16: 125–46.

West Midlands Health (1994) *Spotlight on Primary Care*, Birmingham: West Midlands Regional Health Authority.

Chapter 8

Local authorities servicing health
Rediscovering an historic role

Simon Sedgwick-Jell

INTRODUCTION

Because local government now provides a myriad range of services, it is easy to overlook the fact that the origins of modern local government in the middle of the last century lay very much with a concern for public health and perhaps particularly with the health problems caused by inequality. However, we are now at a point after 150 years, when local authorities are once again both wanting and being able to refocus on contributing to redressing health inequalities (Association of Metropolitan Authorities 1994).

By the 1840s, as Britain entered a phase of mature industrialization, something like half the population lived in towns – a proportion which would steadily rise with a disproportionate growth in the largest cities and conurbations. Attendant on this process were staggering levels of urban squalor. Virtually no major town had proper drainage, few even had a remotely safe waste supply. The result was chronic ill health among the lower classes, a burden on the funds available for Poor Relief and the danger for the middle classes that they too could be affected by epidemics that were no respecters of the crude distinctions within the Victorian class system. It is in this context that the Public Health Act of 1848 was enacted, erecting nearly 700 local Boards of Health charged with the responsibility for providing water and drainage systems for local communities, with particular emphasis being put on those where death rates were high. In all major communities these tasks became central to the operations of municipal councils, which themselves had been modestly reformed in 1835. A Public Health Act of 1875 further refined and consolidated the new arrangements, although confusions and anomalies continued to exist for some time to come (Stoker 1989).

As local government increasingly extended the range of its activities in the post-1900 period, one can still see a focus not only on health but also on the particular plight of the disadvantaged. Two examples will suffice. Municipal housing replacements for the decaying, overcrowded slums dating back to the earlier years of the century, had begun to emerge in the late Victorian period. It became, however, a much more significant and universal concern of local government through a series of Acts passed in the years immediately succeeding the First World War. The provision of adequate, modern and hence healthier accommodation for the working classes would now become the jewel in the crown of many progressive authorities (Malpass and Murie 1994). Some of the same trends could be seen in the field of education, initially somewhat patchily, but then comprehensively pulled together in the 1944 Education Act, with its emphasis on such overtly health-orientated developments as a Schools' Medical Service and the provision of school meals with the clear intention of improving children's health through making available to all a scientifically thought-out balanced diet (Deakin 1994).

If, however, we look at the next half-century, a concern for health, let alone a desire to combat inequality, seems to bulk less large in the minds of local authorities. One obvious reason was the creation of a National Health Service separate and distinct from local government structures, though until recently there were at least some formal links between the two sectors, through local authority nominees to the different tiers of the Health Authority. One must also be aware of how local authorities, particularly after the 1974 reorganization of local government in which community health services were transferred to the NHS (Hogg 1991), expanded other functions. Higher education, personal social services, leisure and economic development all became central to the concerns of many of the most progressive authorities. While, notoriously, slum clearance continued and Environmental Health departments continued to grow, the old, focused concern on health issues *per se* seemed to be just one of a huge number of strands woven into the fabric of an increasingly diverse, sophisticated and managed local government structure (Byrne 1994). Local authorities do now have a lead role in providing community care (NHS and Community Care Act 1990), the possibilities and problems of which are discussed elsewhere in this volume. Nevertheless, this has not represented a specific brief with accompanying resources, to concentrate on preventive, public health work, addressing social inequalities (Association of Metropolitan Authorities 1994).

Now, however, we may be at a new turning point. The last two decades have been characterized by a systematic assault on local government through financial mechanisms: notably the capping of council budgets by central dictat and through the creation of a bewildering range of quangos, to deliver services previously democratically controlled by local councils (Davis and Stewart undated). However, within local government, ways are being found to transcend these very obvious impediments.

A growing number of local authorities no longer see themselves simply as direct service providers (Local Government Management Board 1993). But whilst some authorities have divested themselves of traditional local authority responsibilities by contracting these out to the market sector, others see themselves as having a key role to play in community governance – as representing and articulating the needs of their communities across a broad range of sectors including health. Authorities adopting such an approach include Kirklees, which, for example, now has scrutiny commissioners to examine the implications for local people of issues which lie outside local authority traditional responsibilities. A recent instance of their work concerns inquiries into the rate of water disconnections within the borough (Allison and Hartley 1994).

A third group of authorities see their primary role as developing and empowering local communities to articulate their needs directly to other local agencies (Local Government Management Board 1993).

For those authorities who see themselves as having a role in local governance and/or empowering the local community, there is a growing recognition of the interconnections between inequality, poor health, the microenvironment and the changing nature of the world of work. The fight to combat inequality in health is becoming a mainstream concern of these councils up and down the land. They are employing innovative and holistic approaches to this end, even if sometimes only in an enabling rather than in a providing role (Gyford 1991).

This chapter discusses the attempt to incorporate initiatives with clear consequences for reducing health inequalities, in the work of one council: Cambridge City Council (a council which has district powers as well). It concentrates on reviewing three areas – housing policy, transport policy and competitive contract tendering. The author was leader of the council between 1990 and late 1994, during which time the council adopted both a new corporate strategy and a Citizen's Charter, which included as key corporate objectives the aspirations 'to create a clear, safe and healthy City, and to act locally to enhance the global environment' and 'to concentrate on the welfare of the poorest and most disadvantaged in the community' (Cambridge Citizen's Charter 1991). What follows indicates both the possibilities and the frustrations inherent in local government action at a time when the attitude of central government is, intellectually, organizationally and financially, highly unsupportive to innovative local measures designed to counter the impact of social inequalities on health.

Housing policy and warmth

A very marked feature of the Thatcher/Major years in government – 1979 to the present – has been the sea-change in housing policy. A combination of Right to Buy legislation, massive cutbacks in capital funds made available for the provision of public housing and the driving up of rents to so-called market levels has ensured, first, that most local authorities are only housing those in the most desperate circumstances, and second, that a majority of local authority tenants are in receipt of state benefits and are often wholly dependent on them (Boelat 1989). For people facing these conditions life is a constant series of impossible choices – food or warmth, clothes for the children or getting the washing machine repaired. Stress levels are high, and health suffers in adults and children (Blackburn 1993). What should a local authority response be to this situation, in political as well as polemical terms?

An obvious possibility lies in an environmental and energy audit of its own housing stock with the aim of first pinpointing the scale and nature of energy loss and then rectifying the situation by improving insulation, regarding double glazing as a standard feature and replacing high-cost heating systems with those that are most economical to run. Such an approach can significantly benefit tenants financially and lead to a decrease in, notably, bronchial complaints (Elliott and Houston 1993; Quick and Wilkinson 1991). In such diverse cities as Leicester and Cambridge, and increasingly else-where, an approach which seeks to integrate health issues and other policy areas can be seen as attempting to make an appreciable impact on the health, disposable income and quality of life of local residents (Martin and Kadwell 1994).

Cambridge, for example, adopted a comprehensive energy efficiency strategy for its housing stock in 1992. The aims of the programme included the aim 'to provide all tenants with affordable warmth in order to combat fuel poverty and associated health problems' as well as to reap other environmental and financial advantages. By the year 2000 all council houses would have an average National Home Energy Rating of six and all new building would be planned to be rated at at least eight (on a scale of 0–10, 10 being the optimum level). Integral to the scheme was a systematic input from tenants, via the Tenants' Participation Scheme, so that the tenants themselves played a key role in prioritizing the order in which estates benefited from the capital works required. In some cases the results of the programme have a dramatic effect – a complete energy efficiency refurbishment of 'Unity Houses', system-built properties dating from the 1960s, may have cost nearly £20,000 per dwelling but has delivered energy savings of up to £500 per year. The consequences in terms of improved health for low-income tenants is very clear (Rickaby Thompson Associates 1995).

Traffic and health

The example above is, perhaps, an obvious one, but a local council, if both politically brave enough and corporately intelligent enough to take an overall, rather than a piecemeal view of its functions, powers, responsibilities and opportunities can be innovative in the struggle to redress health inequalities. The mounting evidence of the deleterious effects of rising traffic levels on people's health may be well documented and understood but it has yet to be addressed in anything except the most limited of ways (National Society for Clean Air and Environmental Pollution 1992). And again there is a clear link between inequality and health. It is by and large the case that it is not the wealthiest who live in the areas of greatest traffic concentrations, whose children's schools have playgrounds adjacent to main roads or whose houses suffer from a lack of environmentally safe garden space. A local authority that mounted an all-out assault on the assumption that everyone has the right to drive without let or hindrance, could, in time, have a significant impact on an improvement in health. Policies to induce motorists to use 'park and ride' schemes, systematically banning or very severely restricting traffic in an ever-increasing number of areas, deliberately making life easier for cyclists and pedestrians, while making it more difficult for motorists, would undoubtedly be greeted with squeals of pain and outrage on the part of many of the car-owning democracy, but would provide a significant improvement in the quality of life and health for many inner-city inhabitants who are the sufferers from, rather than the owners of cars.

But the emphasis on political bravery is, of course, crucial. Very large numbers of people are now aware of the health risks associated with the over-crowded urban road network in this country. They know that unleaded petrol is somewhat less harmful than leaded, that all cars pollute; some may even do something about it in their own terms – equip their cars with catalytic converters or switch to unleaded fuel. What they will not do willingly, in the main, is to accept a radical change in their own habits and abandon the use of their cars, a move which is deemed to be massively inconvenient even when other means of transport are available – as within towns they almost invariably are. Most politicians quail when confronted with an electorate for whom other people's cars are, yes, perhaps a problem, but their own are sacred symbols of success, ease and independence. But lessons from the past suggest that it could be by focusing on the health issues associated with motor vehicles, that one could begin the process of conversion to a more rational attitude, while disproportionately bettering more disadvantaged groups.

One reason why progressive local authorities devote significant resources to pollution monitoring is to awake their populations as a whole to the very significant health risks attached to air pollution associated with traffic flow. Yes, monitoring will tend to show that the worst pollution is experienced in the more disadvantaged areas, but these are streets which the more affluent, and, perhaps more significantly, their children at least have to traverse. So an argument can be mounted that highly restrictive policies in the field of traffic management, while improving health most for disadvantaged groups in the population, are certainly also going to improve things for other groups as well. Just as working-class smokers have, somewhat grudgingly, come to accept smoke-free buildings because they know it to be actually more healthy, so middle-class motorists could, as a result of consistent and forceful campaigning, come to accept severe restrictions on the erstwhile freedom to drive anywhere regardless of the environmental consequences. The same approach would, of course, be apposite for the most obvious form of ill health associated with traffic accidents. Recent research has indicated that children and adults from working-class backgrounds are statistically the most likely victims of traffic accidents (Quick and Wilkinson 1991), but this does not mean that those less likely to be involved, but still with the potential to be so, could not be convinced of the imperative need for traffic calming measures, lower speed limits and the whole panoply of other policies which can significantly address the carnage which so often seems to be taken for granted.

Again, Cambridge provides a helpful example of how this approach can operate. From the early 1980s the council has been committed to a comprehensive 'park and ride' scheme as a key element in improving the health and environmental quality of, particularly, inner-city areas. In addition; the council carries out pollution monitoring of carbon monoxide, nitrogen oxides and sulphur dioxide, which is now regularly reported in the local press as well as via the publications of community organizations (Cambridge City Council 1994a). After years of frustration the council moved towards a more proactive campaigning and facilitation role. In 1992 a Green Forum was set up, facilitated by the council, but involving community groups, local environmental organizations and concerned individuals. Regular open and delegate meetings helped not only to order the council's priorities, but also to enable health- and environment-oriented information to be disseminated across the wider community. This was with the overt aim of slowly but surely building up a climate of opinion that would support action for health, of which the most obvious example would be to decrease people's emotional commitment to their own cars.

Whether one looks at issues like housing or the management of traffic, it is obvious that what a local authority can achieve in delivering better health to disadvantaged groups is, at least in part, powerfully dependent on the availability of financial resources. Given a current regime of extreme restriction on councils' abilities to determine their own levels of expenditure (Leach et al. 1994), this clearly means that central government attitudes need to change – either to allow local authorities to set the budget they like, as long as they can deal with the inevitable political consequences, or by the straightforward provision of more grant aid to enable redistributive programmes to be implemented. This is not a scenario which it would be wise to view optimistically given the experiences of the last two decades. It is also the case, and one that needs to be mercilessly exposed, that whether one looks at the local government level or at the workings of the national state, there has been a conspicuous absence of an approach to public expenditure that takes or applies the concept of cost benefits in a holistic, cross-sectional manner. The tyranny of short-termism and narrow perspectives has, in the experience of our council, resulted, for example, in the Department of Transport being loath to grant additional resources for a traffic restriction scheme even if over a ten-year period this could have led to fewer accidents, fewer visits to GPs for skin and asthmatic complaints and other knock-on effects (Cambridgeshire County Council 1994a). The lack of integration of central government activities has recently even been acknowledged by the Government itself – through the creation of integrated regional offices, combining the activities of the Department of Trade and Industry, Environment, Transport and Employment. But notably the Department of Health is not included (personal communication Local Government Centre, University of Warwick).[1]

This lack of integration in central government policies can be seen to have a negatively passive effect on the health of the nation, but there is another area which demonstrates that positive actions taken by central government can directly damage the health of a specific group of more disadvantaged workers.

Compulsory competitive tendering and employees' health

One of the cornerstones of Conservative local government policy since 1979 has been the doctrine of CCT – compulsory competitive tendering. Starting from the assumption of public sector inefficiency and the supposed superiority of private sector organizations, huge areas of local authority activities have been opened up to competition (Walsh 1993). Local authorities have proved to be remarkably successful in continuing to provide in-house services – at least among those councils not ideologically hell-bent on shedding as much direct service provision as possible (Walsh 1991). However, there has been a very significant cost to be paid in terms of health, particularly among manual workers who were the first groups to be exposed to the rigours of the unbridled capitalist market place. In order to win contracts in-house, even progressive councils tended to mirror the private sector in looking to major economies in their operations as they prepared the tenders that would pit them against the private sector (Walsh 1991). While, clearly, some of this could represent good housekeeping and the rectification of previous unhelpful inefficiencies, there is another, more malign side. An emphasis on productivity is not necessarily conducive to the maintenance of good health. Municipal labour forces very often have a skewed age profile with many operatives being in their forties and fifties. A group such as street sweepers or garbage collectors, for example, can now find that the demands of CCT are so onerous that they confront the choice between giving up their employment or experiencing successive periods of illness. The social costs of this are obviously very great. Workers with few skills and, hence, of doubtful re-employability are coerced into either continuous ill health, or unemployment, or early retirement, at considerable cost to the state, all of which significantly outweighs the rather marginal savings that CCT exercises increasingly throw up. Such is the illogical way in which a devotion to market forces can seem to operate.

Councils as political bodies can, of course, attempt to have CCT legislation redrawn in the hope that modification, if not outright repeal (unlikely in almost all the probable political circumstances) will help to undo the worst consequences for vulnerable members of the workforce. However, local authorities also need to think of the possibilities for ameliorative action in their role as employers. Here, there is double opportunity and benefit. By, for example, developing, as Cambridge has done, a comprehensive and robust occupational health programme, a council can have a marked impact on the health of its own employees, particularly perhaps those in manual grades (Cambridge City Council 1992). Its occupational health strategy, adopted in 1992 and regularly revised since then, came at a time when the rigours of the CCT process had led to significant redundancies, extra pressure on the remaining workforce in simple physical terms and of course stress for all, as each contract came up for competition. The strategy tried to deal with all these areas, whether by manual handling courses for the two hundred or so still involved in heavy lifting, in-house physiotherapy and free opportunities for physical exercise on the one hand; to stress management courses, alcohol awareness programmes and financial incentives for aspirant non-smokers to wear nicotine patches, on the other. Judging by the lower rate of absences from illness and a drop in ill health retirement (Cambridge City Council 1994b), the strategy seems to indicate that such a programme can significantly improve workers' health and often prolong an active working life among late middle-aged employees, at a time when, as already alluded to, this is a particularly vulnerable group. But also, as a high profile and large local employee, as almost all local authorities will be, a council can establish itself as an exemplar of best practice in this area and actively seek to disseminate information and ideas to the private sector. Two-way exchanges of practice are becoming increasingly common through the plethora of partnerships which local authorities are developing with the private sector as in the case of economic development (Roberts *et al.* 1995).

The scope of local authority initiatives

Almost all local authorities now see themselves as fulfilling a dual role, as direct providers of services and as enablers, utilizing their position at the centre of a spider's web of community life to encourage things to happen in partnership with other agencies, interest groups and even individuals. The balance between the roles clearly differs markedly from authority to authority, often, but by no means invariably, governed by the political style and affiliation of the given local authority, but a basic acceptance of the model is now virtually universal in local government (Roberts *et al.* 1995).

Both approaches can have implications for action on health and inequality. Examples are legion, with a subtly different mix in each particular case. As increasingly the providers of housing for some of the poorest and most vulnerable groups in the community, local authority housing managers and particularly estate offices can often find themselves at the sharp end of problems associated with psychiatric illnesses. Both their own training and awareness and the creation of structures that enable them easily to network with colleagues in both social services and the community psychiatric services can have a favourable impact not only on the health of tenants experiencing such ill health, but also on that of their neighbours. If an authority is going to prioritize the integration into the community of tenants with a variety of health problems, physical and mental, it also has to accept a programme for the active management of a number of potential issues. A good example comes from the area of noise control. To one tenant very loud music can be a significant release from stress, to her or his neighbour it can be a highly significant cause of stress. It is therefore not too far-fetched, given what we know about the most significant causes of stress within a community, to suggest that the establishment of a comprehensive noise-monitoring service, with close links to either an in-house or a voluntary sector mediation service, can be not insignificant in arresting stressful situations which in the past have often been treated in ways that could lead to high levels of dependency on prescribed drugs.

Whatever range of approaches an individual authority takes, a value-added perspective would seem to be essential, but it is only of value if conceptualized broadly and imaginatively. For example, reducing one's housing management costs may be a highly tempting option for an inward-looking authority, particularly given the potential impact on rent levels. However, this can create more problems than it solves for both tenants and the managers themselves, and can also, by, for example, increasing the call on the health service and social services, add to these other agency costs, and with knock-on effects elsewhere in the community.

There can also be more direct financial value-added calculations for local authorities to carry out. If the assumption is made that one of the dominant causes of ill health among disadvantaged groups is a simple lack of money, any action that increases the income of such groups is likely to have a beneficial effect on health. The provision of a comprehensive benefits advice service, directly or indirectly provided, would normally be assumed to bring back into the community, in terms of extra benefits received, between five and ten times the cost of such a service. Money from the general funds of an authority can therefore be deployed in such a way as to benefit directly and disproportionately the most disadvantaged (*Birmingham Voice* 1994; Cambridge Benefits Advice Centre 1994).

CONCLUSIONS

Local authorities can, as both providers and enablers, return to their origins and see health as at the centre of their concerns and responsibilities. Furthermore, if they embrace wholeheartedly innovative, radical and collaborative service-delivering mechanisms they can play a not insignificant role in redressing the balance between health and inequality.

NOTE

1 I should like to thank Steve Martin, Principal Research Fellow, the Local Government Centre, University of Warwick, for advice and help with additional background material for this chapter.

REFERENCES

Allison, C. and Hartley, J. (1994) *The Changing Role of the Corporate centre in Kirklees Metropolitan Council*, Coventry Local Government Centre: University of Warwick.

Association of Metropolitan Authorities (1994) *Local Authorities and Health Services: The Future Role of Local Authorities in the Provision of Health Services*, London: Association of Metropolitan Authorities.

Birmingham Voice (1994) Wednesday 9 March, Issue no. 4, Birmingham: Council Communications Unit.

Blackburn, C. (1993) 'Making poverty a practice issue', *Health and Social Care* 1 (6): 297–305.

Boelat, M. (1989) 'Housing' in Jackson, P. and Terry, F. (eds) *Public Domain*, London: Peat Marwick.

Byrne, T. (1994) *Local Government in Britain, Everyone's Guide to How it Works*, Harmondsworth: Penguin.

Cambridge Benefits Advice Centre (1994) *Annual Report*, Cambridge: Cambridge Benefits Advice Centre.

Cambridge City Council (1991) *Cambridge Citizen's Charter*, Cambridge: Cambridge City Council.

—— (1992) *Occupational Health Strategy*, Cambridge: Cambridge City Council.

—— (1993) *City Services: Annual Report*, Cambridge: Cambridge City Council.

—— (1994a) *Air Pollution in Cambridge*, Cambridge: Cambridge City Council.

—— (1994b) *City Services: Annual Report*, Cambridge: Cambridge City Council.

Davis, H. and Stewart, J. (undated) *The Growth of Government by Appointment: Implications for Local Democracy*, Luton: Local Government Management Board.

Deakin, N. (1994) *The Politics of Welfare*, Hertfordshire: Harvester Wheatsheaf.

Elliott, J. and Houston, J. (1993) *Poverty in Cambridge*, Cambridge: Cambridge City Council.

Gyford, J. (1991) *Citizens, Consumers and Councils*, London: Macmillan.

Hogg, C. (1991) *Healthy Change: Towards Equality in Health*, London: Socialist Health Association.

Leach, S., Stewart, T. and Walsh, K. (1994) *The Changing Organisation and Management of Local Government*, London: Macmillan.

Local Government Management Board (1993) *Fitness for Purpose – Shaping New Patterns of Organisation and Management*, Luton: Local Government Management Board.

Malpass, P. and Murie, A. (1994) *Housing Policy in Practice*, London: Macmillan.

Martin, S. and Kadwell, C. (1994) *The Local Authority and Economic Regeneration in the Mid 1990s: Coordination Community Involvement and Partnership*, Luton: Local Government Management Board.

National Health Service and Community Care Act (1990), London: HMSO.

National Society for Clean Air and Environmental Pollution (1992) *Air Pollution and Human Health*, Brighton: National Society for Clean Air and Environmental Pollution.

Quick, A. and Wilkinson, R. (1991) *Income and Health*, London: Socialist Health Association.

Rickaby Thompson Associates (1995) *Review of Housing Energy Efficiency Strategy*, Cambridge: Rickaby Thompson Associates.

Roberts, V., Russells, H., Harding, A. and Parkinson, M. (1995) *Public, Private, Voluntary Partnerships in Local Government*, Luton: Local Government Management Board.

Stoker, G. (1989) *The Politics of Local Government*, London: Macmillan.

Walsh, K. (1991) *Competitive Tendering for Local Authority Services, Initial Experiences*, London: HMSO.

—— (1993) *Competition and Service – The Impact of the Local Government Act 1988*, London: HMSO.

Chapter 9

Beyond 'us and them'

Trade unions and equality in community care for users and workers

Mick Carpenter

INTRODUCTION: TOWARDS USER-CENTRED AND WORKER-FRIENDLY HEALTH CARE

In this chapter, I address two inseparable areas of concern for those who would wish to promote greater equality in health: the welfare of employed workers and the broader politics of 'user centred' health care provision. I particularly want to revive interest in what appears to have become an unfashionable topic in critical analyses of health and welfare: the progressive possibilities of public service trade unions advancing both the interests of state workers and those who use services. I support the view that the needs and interests of users and carers should be at the centre of discussions about the future of the public health care services. However, there is a danger that, with a growth of 'consumerism', we will not look at employed workers as people with rights and needs, and this holds implications for their own health which humane and effective public services ought to address, but simply regard their labour as a means to the more important end of empowering users. This, indeed, is how government policies now increasingly lead to them being treated. Not only is this unjust and inequitable, with negative effects on the health and well-being of employed health workers, it is also self-defeating. The interests of users and carers cannot in the end be served by the subordination and downgrading of pay and conditions of employed health workers through an alliance between managerialism and consumerism. While reconciling worker–user interests will not be easy, there are alternative ways forward which give priority to the needs and wishes of users but also take those of employed health workers seriously; which are, in other words, 'user-centred and worker-friendly'. Indeed I will show that initiatives along these lines have been developed since the mid-1980s by public service unions like UNISON.

I shall focus on community care in Britain. It is an important and neglected area of health provision and at the cutting edge of debates about how public services can be made more accountable to those who use them. The user movement in this context is also perhaps one of the most significant and encouraging political developments in health and social services since the 1980s. It sees community care as a site for challenging narrow, biomedical approaches to disability and care which define people as either in need of cure, or management and control, by articulating an alternative agenda of empowerment and autonomy. If government-sponsored consumerism constructs this agenda in largely individualist terms, in ways that pitch users against employed workers, it becomes an urgent necessity to show how user and employed worker interests can be reconciled, and to demonstrate that the pursuit of a more equal experience of health is an issue that transcends 'user'/'worker' divides.

FROM TRADITIONAL TO 'NEW' PUBLIC SERVICE UNIONISM

In the 1970s the rapid growth of trade unionism among welfare state workers was regarded by some analysts as one of the most hopeful developments since the creation of the post-war welfare state. James O'Connor (1973), for example, recognized that there was a growing 'fiscal crisis' of the state and that public aspirations for social welfare spending were expanding beyond the ability of the capitalist state to finance them. The welfare state would either be restructured to provide a better fit with capitalist accumulative interests, or shift in a genuinely socialist direction through a progressive alliance between working-class users and unionized public sector workers. O'Connor's was just one of a number of Marxian analyses of the time in which discussions of public sector trade unionism were accorded a central place (for example, see also Gough 1979).

One thing often missing from these structural theories, however, was much discussion of how health and welfare services were experienced at a day to day level by those who used them and the mixed feelings that might arise from interventions by state workers in people's personal lives. One of the innovative features of feminist analyses of the welfare state is that they viewed welfare state intervention as having an *inherently contradictory* impact at the micropolitical level of daily life. Thus Elizabeth Wilson (1977) was one of the first to argue that the welfare state at one and the same time 'helped' women but on terms which reinforced patriarchal dependency and oppression. The implications of this emerging analysis was that it was necessary to transform the day to day workings of the welfare state itself so that people did not experience it as something 'over' them. The most elaborated attempt to develop this approach was by the London–Edinburgh Weekend Return Group (1979). In a pamphlet published in the wake of the 1978–9 'Winter of Discontent' – involving widespread strike action by public service workers – they recognized the potentially divisive effects of conflicts of interest between public sector workers and users of services and offered a sober analysis of how negative experiences of state services had fuelled it. On the more optimistic side, they spelled out means by which unions were seeking to develop forms of action which hit management but did not harm users, while at the same time advocating joint action between welfare state workers and users to 'prefigure' more progressive forms of state intervention.

These suggestions were made more than fifteen years ago. It is hard to think of a significant comparable analysis since, though in fact public service unions themselves have been actively developing practical means of bridging this divide. This chapter therefore seeks to return to these issues. It draws on the author's experience of working with public sector unions since the 1970s, particularly those that combined to form UNISON in 1993 as the largest union in Britain, through the coming together of the Confederation of Health Service Employees (COHSE), the National Union of Public Employees (NUPE), and the National and Local Government Officers' Association (NALGO).

THATCHERISM AND THE PROMOTION OF WELFARE INDIVIDUALISM

What could not have been predicted in the 1970s was how the Thatcher and Major governments have managed to restructure British welfare capitalism within the framework of a parliamentary democracy in ways contrary to the interests of large numbers of ordinary people and often unpopular with them. This has been partly due to the electoral system, for, however unpopular between elections, it was possible periodically to 'legitimize' minority Conservative governments (in terms of votes cast). At the same time, concerted efforts were made to construct a state structure immune from continuous popular pressure, by curtailing the democratic powers of local government bodies and setting up a multitude of unaccountable quangos. As part of this strategy, individual consumerism in public services was encouraged to a limited degree because it was thought to be a means of building an alliance between users and managers against state workers and (where relevant) local politicians. The public sector strikes in the 1970s had had the effect of underlining the contradictory nature of people's 'need' for public service: they made people feel vulnerable by withdrawing something they relied on, while at the same time stirring up negative feelings they had about what was normally on offer to them. The nature of welfare services, whether organized according to bureaucratic rules (like council housing) or professional discretion (like health care and social services), was that any citizenship rights *to* services were not usually matched by many significant rights *within* them. Thus they were based on imposed conceptions of 'need'.

Conservative welfare individualism sought as far as possible to prise open these divisions between state workers and users. Where wholesale privatization was not politically feasible, state services were reorganized in ways that appeared to offer a 'new deal' to users, for the lack of responsiveness was portrayed, with some justification, as the result of services that had previously been 'provider led'. A central feature of this new strategy was a combination of more coercive management strategies for dealing with state workers and contracting out of publicly funded services, which Hunter (1993) appropriately calls the 'new public management'. It was particularly associated with Sir Roy Griffiths' efforts to reorganize public services, including community care, as if they were competitive retail businesses which would thereby yield both greater 'efficiency' *and* improvements for users (as customers), through a management–consumer alliance (Griffiths 1988).

TRADE UNION RESPONSES

Part of the reason why the Thatcher and Major Governments have not pursued a policy of wholesale privatization of health and social services is that public service unions have mobilized their members and the wider public to prevent it. Thus, in 1983, the first Thatcher Government had to back-track on the leaked 'Think Tank' proposals, which showed that the Cabinet were thinking of introducing a programme of wholesale privatization of wide areas of health and welfare, including the National Health Service. In the ensuing public furore they realized that 'public opinion' was not ready for such a frontal assault on the welfare state. They learnt that they needed instead to pursue their long-term intentions in a more piecemeal way. Hence they decided to pursue a combination of creeping privatization and new public management approaches which have ostensibly sought to 'improve' rather than to undermine public services. Yet the goal of pushing privatization to the currently feasible limit has always figured prominently, and one 'reform' has always been succeeded by others. It is certainly the case that unions have found it harder to mobilize public support against this more incremental and politically sophisticated approach.

It is important to remember that in seeking to build counter-alliances with users, trade unions have not entirely abandoned traditional forms of action. That strikes have been less frequent may be due less to a concern not to alienate public support, than to the combined coercive effects of unemployment, job insecurity and draconian anti-union legislation. Even so, there have been some significant campaigns of industrial action in the public services since the mid-1980s, including national actions by teachers, nurses, ambulance workers, rail workers, and a considerable number of local disputes involving a wide variety of public service employees. Many have enjoyed considerable popular support, though this has not often been sufficient in itself to ensure success in the face of an obdurate government. Despite this, and certainly compared to the rest of the trade union movement, public service unions have weathered the last fifteen years reasonably well. Much of this is due to the fact that the employment base in the public services has until recently remained relatively intact. This, in turn, is in part attributable to the emergence of a 'new' public service unionism, seeking to develop new ways of pursuing grievances which maximize publicity and difficulty for the government, while minimizing disruption to users of services, in order to mobilize public support.

In seeking to build alliances between employed workers and users against the government, the most important aim has been to create a 'community' of interest by showing that the pursuit of efficiency and cost-cutting will not only lead to deterioration of pay and employment conditions, but also to a decline in the quality of service, for example, that contracting out of hospital cleaning services will lead to lower standards and increase the risk of cross-infection. On the whole, unions have often won the arguments, but been defeated by a government cushioned by an electoral system which has enabled it to drive through unpopular measures. Nevertheless, numerous campaigns have demonstrated the ability of unions to construct such alliances (Carpenter 1994), and in the process a formidable degree of experience and expertise has been developed. These have included campaigns against contracting out of hospital cleaning services and the privatization of water companies in the 1980s, against the health service 'reforms' in the 1990s and, perhaps most successful of all, the Union of Communication Workers' campaign which helped to force the Major Government in 1994 to shelve plans to privatize the Post Office (at least by direct means). Were it not for these campaigns, the health and welfare services themselves might have been more extensively privatized, for the Government has known in advance that their proposals will elicit strong opposition. Even when monopoly utilities like gas and water have been privatized, workers, through UNISON and other unions, have continued to call the government to account for empty promises that the market would lead to improvements for users, when it has instead led to large increases in user charges and disconnections for those unable to pay them, to help finance profits for shareholders and the phenomenal salaries and other perks of higher management (Carpenter 1994). Public service unions, therefore, remain a significant source of resistance and continuing challenge to the inegalitarian effects of government policies.

The new public service unionism has, however, achieved more than the necessary exposure of the negative features of Conservative policies and a check upon government power. Unions like UNISON have also recognized the need to respond to the government's restructuring of the welfare state by addressing the oppressive and sometimes abusive features of health and welfare services in the past and constructing alternative visions of how public services could be organized in future. The chief lesson to have emerged from these efforts is the need to defend citizenship rights to well funded and universal health and welfare services, while at the same time seeking to make these more responsive to the needs and wishes of individuals and groups. Despite the claims made for it, the individualist consumerism associated with new public management approaches is not up to this task. It is true that we are unique individuals, but our individuality is shaped by the social context of our lives and their structuring by 'race', gender, class, age and other divisions. We need individually appropriate services which take account of these social dimensions. Since consumerism only recognizes the atomized individual decision maker, divorced from their social context, it is apparent that it does not seek to empower everyone equally. It is also based on a simplistic 'zero sum' notion of power which sees *either* the consumer *or* the producer as sovereign. Hence the challenge is to find ways of developing schemes of *joint* empowerment of users and employees at all levels within democratically organized and decentralized public services, as alternatives to bureaucratic, professional and managerial forms of domination. The most serious deficiency of the consumer model, however, is its failure to recognize that users and carers are actually *producers of health and welfare* and need to be empowered as active participants within the health and welfare labour process, not just as passive consumers.

What I call 'user-centred and worker-friendly' community care seeks to develop these social and democratic principles systematically out of a critique of the Conservative Government's approach, drawing inspiration from some of the sophisticated campaigns developed by UNISON and its predecessor unions since the 1980s. I now wish to illustrate how these have been pursued in response to the Government's community care policies.

THE EXAMPLE OF COMMUNITY CARE

The origins and effects of the 1990 NHS and Community Care Act are complex. In its essentials, however, it fits firmly within the new public management model described here, involving a contradictory attempt to ration services in order to achieve savings, while at the same time building a consumerist constituency of user empowerment against employed workers. By being aware of the tensions between these two aims, an alternative 'community care alliance' can be built which unites employed workers, users and carers in the campaign for well funded, 'user-centred and worker-friendly' services.

On the one hand, the new system designed for the Government by Sir Roy Griffiths was designed to cap expenditure and shift the costs of caring for the health and well-being of increasing numbers of older people on to them and their families. By the end of the 1980s the Conservatives were concerned about the extent to which they had subsidized the growth of social security payments for private residential care to the tune of more than £1 billion, compared to £10 million in 1979 (Local Government Information Unit 1990). They were also seeking to rationalize the health service by reducing psychiatric beds, which fell 44 per cent from 1979 to 1992 while only minimal gestures were made towards resourcing alternatives in the community (Eaton 1994). Finally, they were seeking to transfer the responsibility for the long-term care of older people out of the NHS by redefining it as 'social' rather than 'health' care (Carlisle 1995).

On the other hand, however, while favouring a 'family' model of care *by* the community, Griffiths clearly recognized that some input by the Government was necessary. Surprisingly he also endorsed the 'normal living' or 'normalization' principles which had come out of the radical users' movements of the 1970s as a framework for intervention. Normalization strategies are optimistic in that they seek to provide supportive services to empower users to leave institutions and participate in society on their own terms, based on the correct supposition that institutional care as currently organized by state services is often anti-therapeutic (Brown and Smith 1992).

The essential elements of Griffiths' approach became law in 1990, though full implementation of the financial provisions had to wait until April 1993. In theory a right to services to make 'normal living' feasible was now possible through assessment of individual needs and the provision of appropriate 'packages' of care. Services would be made accountable to users at both the individual and collective level of local community care planning. To the surprise of many, local government was given the 'lead' responsibility for this new system. Yet as is now rapidly becoming apparent, rather than representing a new dawn for users, one quickly responsive to individuals on the basis of need alone, the needs-assessment process is becoming more a set of hurdles which people have to overcome to get such services. A largely automatic right in the past to financial support for residential care has been taken away and new users' needs for both community and residential services are being much more closely scrutinized through bureaucratic procedures of care management. Rather than providing an open-ended commitment to needs-based support for normal living, the Government is simply transferring the social security money in stages to local authorities, where it will only be transitionally ring-fenced, and people's rights to services will also be means-tested for ability to pay. Assuming you pass through all these hurdles, the money to provide you with what you need may just not be there or else there might be local problems of supply (Rickford 1994). All this necessitates other bureaucratic procedures to ration services among different users according to those rated as having the highest 'priority'. From the local authority's financial point of view it makes sense to fund those in most urgent need who may otherwise have to go into expensive residential care. This means that more preventive work with those who currently are not defined as in priority 'need' goes by the board. That this system is, therefore, raising expectations that it cannot deliver is becoming only too apparent, as there are already signs of massive pressures on community care budgets up and down the country, exacerbated by the effects of the NHS internal market, which is leading to the discharge of larger numbers of frail older people from hospitals (various UNISON branches personal communication; Rickford 1994). By the end of 1994 the Association of County Councils estimated that twenty-four local authorities were in serious difficulty. One, the Isle of Wight, had run out of community care funds four months before the end of the year (Gilbert 1995). In many of the local protests against community care cuts, the growing counter-alliance between user groups and trade unions against the Government has been very visible, often in traditionally Conservative strongholds (various UNISON branches personal communication).

The fundamental problem with the new public management approach, underlying these increasing funding difficulties, is its belief in the managerial 'quick fix'. It was either naïvely or cynically believed that all community care provision needed was some minimal financial pump-priming and increased managerial efficiency would do the rest. This would then enable frail people and those with disabilities to lead integrated and independent lives in the community, with ready help being offered from family, friends, neighbours and voluntary groups. Because the Act constructs community care as an individualized commodity there is no recognition of the need to sustain it by government action to support communities. 'Normal living' depends not just on provision of services but access to employment, income, housing, leisure, transport, environmental protection and so on. Not only did Griffiths hardly refer to these, they have all been under threat over the last fifteen years as a result of a steady erosion of public provision and the failure of Government economic policies (Savage and Robins 1990; Lowe 1993).

If community care legislation often has an invidious effect on users and carers, it has also added to pressures on employed workers. The Act stipulates that 85 per cent of transferred funds must be spent in the independent (voluntary and commercial) sector, unfairly denying public sector employees a chance to prove their worth and creating a coercive shift towards privatization of services. As 'street-level bureaucrats' (Lipsky 1980), those remaining in the state sector are increasingly assessment staff, who must work the bureaucracy of needs assessment, means testing and rationing and deal with the frustrations of users and carers, adding to the stress levels upon them. While independent sector services can be equal or superior to those provided by public authorities, it is patently obvious that one of the chief ways that 'efficiency' is being achieved is not by raising standards but by driving down wages and conditions. As Chris May, UNISON's Birmingham voluntary sector spokesperson put it: 'What we have is a statutory sector in which pay and conditions are not that good, we have a voluntary sector which is worse, and a private sector which is horrific.'

He was speaking in the wake of the publication of the Public Services Privatization Research Unit report into pay and conditions in the independent sector which showed that care staff were paid as little as £1.70 an hour, with an average of £3.26 (Linehan 1994). Some of the worst conditions are to be found in the mushrooming domiciliary care agencies which, unlike reputable organizations such as Crossroads, put little emphasis on reasonable working conditions. Local authority home-help hours are being cut and being replaced by agencies which recruit young people and women on extremely low hourly rates, who are given little or no training and may be sent out at night on their own. Nor is there any check made on recruitment and training standards (various UNISON branches personal communication). In short, the coercive shift to privatization which is an integral feature of the 1990 Act, means that community care is becoming casualized as part of the growth of the new service economy of low paid women and young people, to the detriment of both employees and service users. This, in turn, contributes to widening social inequalities, on both sides of the user–provider divide, which have been shown to be so corrosive to the health of those who have lost most from these policies (Quick and Wilkinson 1991).

COMMUNITY CARE AND MENTAL HEALTH

Despite all these problems, unions like UNISON have not waged purely defensive struggles but have supported and campaigned nationally and locally for community care based on principles of 'normal living'. I have documented these efforts in some detail elsewhere (Carpenter 1994). Here I would like to focus mainly on a particularly adventurous initiative.

One area of community care where the Government has shown itself to be both cautious and niggardly has been in the shift of mental health services to the community. Enormous sums of money have been saved by closing down psychiatric beds, very little of which has been used to finance alternative provision (Labour Party 1994). At the same time the Government has sought to maintain a highly medicalized system based on a smaller number of intensively used District General Hospital beds. As this system has run into trouble, the response has been to reinforce a coercive approach focused on 'high risk' individuals. From 1994, stigmatizing 'at risk' registers have been set up to keep a watchful eye on those users who might be perceived to be a threat to themselves or others (Crepaz-Keay 1994). Psychiatry has, therefore, shifted towards an under-resourced 'medical model in the community', which retains medical power and exhibits strong controlling features, rather than a social approach based on normalization principles. Nevertheless a struggle is going on both to increase resources and shift provision in a 'post-medical' direction, in which the mental health users' movement is playing the most prominent part (Rogers *et al.* 1992).

In the past, the trade union movement has often been suspicious of the user movement. For example, psychiatric nurses have often defended an institutional system based on psychiatrists even though they have been subordinated to them. This has been partly to protect their jobs and the way of life that grew up around hospitals, but also because they wanted to defend the powers of control over users delegated to them by psychiatrists. However, in the mid-1980s this started to change when some psychiatric nurse members of COHSE allied themselves with users to protest publicly against the plans to give psychiatrists powers of compulsory supervision of users in the community. This was part of a more general change of heart, whereby the union started to support the closure of traditional mental hospitals and the shift to a social and democratic model in the community (Carpenter 1994).

One exciting outcome of this emerging alliance was the production in 1992 of the COHSE/MIND *Guidelines for Empowering Users of Mental Health Services* (Read and Wallcraft 1992). These involved the union seeking practical help and advice from members of Survivors Speak Out, a radical self-help group, on how employed staff might empower users. The message that comes across loud and clear from the *Guidelines* is that it is possible to empower both users and employees, as hierarchical structures not only oppress users but also demand compliance from staff. As Jim Read and Jan Wallcraft, the authors of the *Guidelines*, put it: 'It is not easy to empower or value others when you do not feel valued and powerful yourself' (Read and Wallcraft 1992: 5).

While recognizing the constraints that workers often face, the *Guidelines* suggest that both individuals and branches can take action to empower users. For example, as individuals, nurses can start to implement principles of 'informed consent' by offering choices rather than imposing treatments, by listening and talking to users and not dismissing complaints and anxieties as symptoms of mental illness. At a more collective level, the *Guidelines* suggest that user empowerment will only work if there is genuine power sharing. This may require the use of facilitators who are or have been users and arrangements for acting on users' expressed preferences. They also suggest models of good practice for involving users in staff appointments. Already some promising attempts have been made within UNISON branches to use the *Guidelines* to develop local schemes of user empowerment, though these have not yet been evaluated (Karen Jennings, UNISON Professional Officer, personal communication). Of course, this is only a beginning, but there has been some useful follow-up work since, in which Jim Read and Jan Wallcraft (1994) have produced joint MIND/UNISON *Guidelines on Advocacy for Mental Health Workers*. These go into more detail about the theory and practice of various types of advocacy and give some examples of how it might be made to work in practice. The examples, drawn from case study materials, include discussion of how an advocate was able to assist 'David' at a care planning meeting prior to discharge, to communicate his wish to reduce his dependence on medication when he leaves hospital and to receive help in doing so. In another instance, the ability of 'citizen advocacy' support provided by volunteers to help 'Jill' realize her desire to stay out of hospital is discussed. At a more collective level, they cite the experience of a users'-only Patients' Council in a mental hospital and their effective protests at a local health authority's decision to build a new mental health unit without consulting either patients or staff. At a national level, they cite the influence of user self-advocacy in campaigning alongside UNISON, the British Association of Social Workers and other organizations against the proposed intro-duction of Community Supervision Orders and the experience of users in presenting an alternative policy of 'crisis cards' to the House of Commons Select Committee investigating the issue (Read and Wallcraft 1994). Alongside this material is advice on how staff may either 'support or sabotage' patients' councils and advocacy projects. For example, it suggests that:

Staff can support advocacy by:

- Arranging or requesting training in advocacy and empowerment for all staff.
- Finding out what advocacy is available locally and passing information on to patients and other staff.
- Treating the advocate, whether paid or unpaid, with the respect you would show to a professional representative such as a solicitor.
- Being prepared to explain to other staff, as many times as necessary, why advocacy is needed.

Staff can sabotage advocacy by:

- Trying to persuade the advocate to support your point of view rather than the patient's.
- Refusing independent advocacy on the grounds that a relative can put the patient's views forward, that everything is fine or that the patient is too confused, or that it makes the patient too powerful and makes your job harder.
- Treating the presence of an advocate as a personal attack on your integrity (see Read and Wallcraft 1994).

Though such a pronounced emphasis on user self-advocacy is admittedly unusual, it is just one example of a larger number of national and local union initiatives aimed at enhancing the position of employed workers, while at the same time improving the quality of service to users. This includes the commitment, for example, that public service unions have given to the development of training in general and National Vocational Qualifications (NVQ) in particular. Public service unions have focused on these schemes, which emerged in the 1980s, because of the opportunity they present to counter the de-skilling and cheapening tendencies of new public management policies, in the hope that they will also lead to improvements in pay and conditions of front line staff and at the same time secure improvements in the quality of services provided.

More directly, to help ensure that greater public recognition was given to users' requirements and that these were influential in shaping union policy, NALGO, in 1992, sponsored qualitative research from the Institute of Public Policy Research on the views of users of community care services. This found widespread endorsement of principles of independent living and that people, whatever the nature and degree of their disability, 'overwhelmingly' wanted to live in the community. Rather than being a cheap option, community care was therefore something which had to be 'made' to work (Mackie 1992). A final example of public service unions placing users' welfare together with that of workers at the centre of their practice is Quality Care, the joint statement by West Midlands COHSE/NALGO/NUPE in 1992, anticipating the formation of UNISON. This pledged a strong commitment to well resourced and democratically organized community care services, accountable to all workers and users, as a basis for its campaigning work around community care.

CONCLUSION: TOWARDS A THIRD WAVE?

It might be regarded as idealistic to see in these developments the beginnings of a 'third wave' in the development of community care, based on user centred and worker friendly principles, which overcomes the deficiencies of both the poorly resourced and paternalistic approach characteristic of the 1960s and 1970s and the disappointed expectations raised by the managerialism and consumerism of the New Right era. Nevertheless there is evidence that this approach could become more influential in the future, if the Labour Party were to regain political power. In 1993, a Labour Party discussion document on community care recognized that, if 'normal living' principles are to succeed, there is a need to provide forms of community care provision that offer genuine empowerment to users and carers. It recognized that the encouragement of advocacy and self-advocacy at the heart of community care provision is necessary to make this possible, together with a shift from the current bureaucratic system of needs assessment. The document also argued that well funded and reorganized community care services are not sufficient and that more egalitarian policies around such issues as housing, employment and income are also required to underwrite health and well-being (Labour Party Discussion Document1993). All this gives grounds for optimism, although the economic circumstances that are likely to face any future Labour government, as well as the current rightwards political drift within the Party, might constrain the extent to which a progressive community agenda of the kind envisaged in this chapter will be implemented. All the more reason, then, to consolidate the emerging employee–user alliance to ensure that community care becomes what it has never been – a central rather than a residual element of public health policy – in ways that meet the interests of both users and employees. All the more reason also, to campaign for services which seek to mitigate rather than exacerbate divisions of 'us versus them' between users, carers and employed workers. We may be on one side or the other of this divide at any particular time in our lives, or we may combine two or all of these roles. By uniting, therefore, in a campaign to place users at the centre of public health care services in ways that address the human needs of *all* those involved in care we are actually, whatever our health care responsibilities at any particular time, campaigning for ourselves.

REFERENCES

Brown, H. and Smith, H. (1992) *Normalisation: A Reader for the Nineties*, London: Routledge.

Carlisle, D. (1995) 'Divided State', *Nursing Times* 15 March: 14–15.

Carpenter, M. (1994) *Normality is Hard Work: Trade Unions and the Politics of Community Care*, London: Lawrence and Wishart.

Crepaz-Keay, D. (1994) 'I wish to Register a Complaint . . . ', *Openmind*, October/November: 5.

Eaton, L. (1994) 'Why is Community Care Failing the Mentally Ill?', *Mental Illness: The Facts*, Supplement to *Community Care* 30 April: 7–9.

Gilbert, J. (1995) 'Ways, But No Means', *Nursing Times* 1 February: 13–14.

Gough, I. (1979) *The Political Economy of the Welfare State*, London: Macmillan.

Griffiths, Sir Roy (1988) *Community Care: An Agenda for Action*, London: HMSO.

Hunter, D. (1993) 'To Market! To Market! A New Dawn for Community Care', *Health and Social Care in the Community* 1 (1): 3–10.

Labour Party (1994) *Health 2000: The Health and Wealth of the Nation in the 21st Century*, London: The Labour Party.

Labour Party Discussion Document (1993) *New Directions in Community Care*, London: The Labour Party.

Linehan, T. (1994) 'Private Pain', *Community Care* 11–17 August: 15–16.

Lipsky, M. (1980) *Street Level Bureaucracy: Dilemmas of the Individual in Public Services*, New York: Russell Sage Foundation.

Local Government Information Unit (1990) *Caring for People – The Government's Plans for Care in the Community*, Special Briefing No. 32.

London–Edinburgh Weekend Return Group (1979) *In and Against the State*, London: Pluto Press.

Lowe, R. (1993) *The Welfare State in Britain Since 1945*, London: Macmillan.

Mackie, L. (1992) *Community Care: Users' Experiences*, London: NALGO.

O'Connor, J. (1973) *The Fiscal Crisis of the State*, New York: St James Press.

Quick, A. and Wilkinson, R.G. (1991) *Income and Health*, London: Socialist Health Association.

Read, J. and Wallcraft, J. (1992) *Guidelines for Empowering Users of Mental Health Services*, Banstead: COHSE/MIND.

—— (1994) *Guidelines on Advocacy for Mental Health Workers*, London: UNISON/MIND.

Rickford, F. (1994) 'The System Grows Frail', *Guardian*, 30 November.

Rogers, A., Pilgrim, D. and Lacey, R. (1992) *Experiencing Psychiatry: Users' Views of Services*, London: Macmillan.

Savage, S. and Robins, L. (1990) *Public Policy Under Thatcher*, London: Macmillan.

Wilson, E. (1977) *Women and the Welfare State*, London: Tavistock.

Part III

Information for change

Chapter 10

Reducing child health inequalities
Insights and strategies for health workers

Nick Spencer

INTRODUCTION

The publication of the Black Report (Townsend and Davidson 1982) in 1980 opened a new period of vigorous debate about the nature, extent and explanations of health inequalities. This chapter draws on some of that recent work as a basis for addressing health inequalities amongst children in the UK. Problems of methodology and interpretation are considered in detail in order to inform the arguments and place them in their political context. Strategies for combating child health inequalities are discussed in the light of this deepened understanding before the chapter concludes by considering implications for future research and the barriers, both political and professional, to working for equality in child health.

UNDERSTANDING HEALTH INEQUALITIES

Limitations of official data

The Black Report drew almost exclusively on the mortality differentials in 'Decennial Supplements on Occupational Mortality' published by the Registrar General's office to demonstrate the extent of health inequalities. The measure of socio-economic status used by these supplements is the Registrar General's Social Class (RGSC) based on the occupation of the male head of the household. This classification has undergone a series of changes since 1911. There are now six classes: SCI (professional); SCII (managerial); SCIIInm (non-manual); SCIIIm (skilled manual); SCIV (semi-skilled manual); SCV (unskilled manual). An unclassified heterogeneous group comprising the unemployed, students, service personnel and lone mothers is sometimes incorporated in official data. Occupation-based measures such as the RGSC have consistently demonstrated health inequalities in the UK (Townsend and Davidson 1982). However, the RGSC has been criticized in recent years on several grounds: there are very wide variations in health outcomes between occupations which make up the same social class (Jones and Cameron 1984); within class income variation is greater than that between classes (Smith *et al*. 1994); the RGSC fails to reflect the fine-grained inequalities between and within occupations (ibid.); the RGSC underestimates the association between social factors and adverse health outcomes (ibid.); the occupation of the male head of household does not accurately reflect the economic experience of women (Oakley *et al*. 1993); and groups such as lone mothers and the unemployed living on state benefit are excluded from the classification (Cooper 1991).

Two other limitations of official data which specifically affect understanding of health inequalities amongst children and young people are also worth detailing. First, perinatal and infant mortality and birth weight data routinely published by the Office for Population Censuses and Surveys (OPCS) use the RGSC but include only births within marriage. Births outside marriage now contribute almost 30 per cent of all UK births and contain some of the most disadvantaged groups (Cooper 1991). Second, official data on health inequalities are largely confined to mortality. The decline in mortality rates, particularly in childhood, renders mortality data less useful in studying health inequalities. These limitations of officially reported data on health inequalities have impeded understanding of the magnitude of health inequalities and have contributed to confusion within the causal debate. However, some important studies have overcome these limitations and thrown valuable light on the magnitude and causes of health inequalities.

Official data reanalysed

The Registrar General's data indicate that inequalities in mortality increased between the early 1950s and the late 1970s (Townsend and Davidson 1982; Pamuk 1988). However, infant mortality seemed to be bucking the trend so that Townsend and Davidson state: 'In the late 1970s the class differences in infant mortality diminished' (p.9). This apparent reduction in inequalities in infant mortality was seen as evidence that the conclusions of the Black Report might be invalid

(Gordon 1986). Reanalysis of social class inequality in infant mortality revealed that this apparent reduction in inequalities disappeared if births outside marriage were included in the analysis (Pamuk 1988). Pamuk (ibid.) uses a relative index of inequality (RII) which shows unchanged levels of inequality throughout the period from 1920 to 1980 (p.13).

Judge and Benzeval (1993) employ a different technique to examine inequalities in child mortality. They linked mortality and census data to derive relative risks of death in various age groups of children in households headed by 'unoccupied' women (women caring for children on state benefits) compared with the conventional RGSCs. The relative risk for death in all age groups is higher in the 'unoccupied' group than Social Class V, especially in the 10–14 year age group.

Alternative measures of socio-economic status to the RGSC

Researchers in the USA have used income as the main measure of socio-economic status but in this country researchers have been reluctant to do so despite Townsend's demonstration that detailed and reliable income data can be obtained (Townsend 1979). Various income proxies have been used which provide alternatives to the RGSC: housing tenure (Oakley *et al.* 1994); car ownership (Smith *et al.* 1994); finely differentiated occupational grades within the Civil Service (Marmot *et al.* 1984), or residence in a house with a garden (Smith *et al.* 1990). Socio-economic indices have been developed which attempt to overcome the limitations of single variable measures by combining variables; for example, Osborn (1987) developed a Social Index based on National Childhood Development Study data. Increasing use has been made in recent years of measures derived from census data which reflect the level of material deprivation in areas of residence. The Jarman Score (Jarman 1983) was one of the first to be used, but has been superseded by more accurate deprivation indices such as the Carstairs (Carstairs and Morris 1992) and Townsend (Townsend *et al.* 1988) indices.

New evidence related to health inequalities using alternative measures

Evidence related to health inequalities in adults has come from two major sources in the UK: the Whitehall Study of civil servants (Marmot *et al.* 1984) and the OPCS Longitudinal Study (Fox *et al.*

1985). In the Whitehall Study of middle-aged male civil servants, employment grade and car ownership contributed independently to mortality risk (Smith *et al.* 1990) with cumulative effects. The addition of an extra marker of socio-economic status, use of a garden, results in a further differentiation with an all-cause mortality of 32/ 1000 person years in clerical staff without a car or a garden compared with 11/1000 person years for administrative staff with a car and garden (Smith *et al.* 1990). Self-perceived ill-health, measured in the second Whitehall Study (Marmot *et al.* 1991), also demonstrated a substantial difference between employment grades. The importance of these findings is that all the civil servants studied would be classified as social class III non-manual or higher in the RG's classification, suggesting that there is a fine-grained gradient in adverse health outcomes closely related to socio-economic status which is not reflected in analyses based on the Registrar General's social classes.

The OPCS longitudinal study has proved particularly valuable in studying the effects of unemployment on health which are poorly examined by occupation-based measures. Analysis of mortality in the 1970s amongst the study's participants showed that unemployment in 1971 was associated with higher than expected mortality and that unemployment itself was much more likely to be experienced during the 1970s by those in the 'lowest' class groups (Fox and Shewry 1988). The wives of men who were unemployed in 1971 also had a higher than expected mortality.

Recent studies from the Northern region of England (Phillimore *et al.* 1994) and Scotland (McLoone and Boddy 1994; McCarron *et al.* 1994) report widening mortality differentials between those living in deprived and affluent areas in the period from the early 1980s to the early 1990s. In the most deprived 20 per cent of electoral wards in the Northern region infant mortality did not fall between the early 1980s and the early 1990s, during which time a substantial fall was noted in the most affluent 20 per cent of wards (Phillimore *et al.* 1994).

A number of other studies have reported health inequalities in childhood:

1 Preliminary results from studies in the West Midlands Health Region (unpublished) show that the relative risk for infants born in the most deprived, compared with the least deprived areas of the region, is 2.23 for stillbirths, 3.42 for neonatal deaths and 2.63

for perinatal deaths. These risks are much higher than those predicted by social class.

2 Hospital admission for bronchiolitis during a major outbreak in the winter of 1989–90 in Sheffield was positively correlated with residence in deprived electoral wards of the city (Spencer *et al.* 1995).

3 Children under the age of two years living in deprived electoral wards in Sheffield in 1980 and 1985 had a significantly higher risk of multiple hospital admission (three or more) for organic causes than children in non-deprived wards (Spencer *et al.* 1993).

4 Similar wide differences between most and least deprived areas were found in studies of height and birth weight in Northumberland (Reading *et al.* 1990).

5 Osborn (1987) showed that the Social Index accounted for more of the variance in children's scores on the English Picture Vocabulary Test, children's anti-social behaviour and depression amongst their mothers, than the same data analysed by RGSC.

Studies of housing and child health (Martin *et al.* 1987), homelessness and health (Royal College of Physicians of London 1994) and nutrition among the poor (National Children's Homes 1991; Dowler and Calvert 1995) have also increased our understanding of the *mechanisms* by which poverty adversely affects the health of mothers and children. The double jeopardy of Black children and their families has been explored in various studies which highlight the dual effects of poverty and racism (Grimsley and Bhat 1986).

International comparisons have also contributed to better understanding of health inequalities, suggesting that inequalities of income distribution may be more significant than gross national product (GNP) (Wilkinson 1989). This is exemplified in both developed and less developed countries where some, such as Costa Rica, Cuba and Sri Lanka, perform much better in health terms than would be expected for their GNP, in part because of more equitable income distribution (United Nations Development Project 1994). Costa Rica, with a GNP per capita of $1,218, now has a life expectancy equivalent to that of the UK, with a GNP per capita of $11,059 (World Health Organization 1995).

METHODOLOGICAL ISSUES IN THE INTERPRETATION OF HEALTH INEQUALITIES DATA

The data presented above represent a major contribution to our understanding of health inequalities. The magnitude and trends in health differentials which they depict are difficult to explain in behavioural terms (Smith *et al.* 1994). However, the causal debate has continued, with individual behaviour still being the main focus of preventive approaches (Department of Health 1992) and some commentators even arguing that health inequalities do not really exist and, if they do, their significance is overrated (Le Fanu 1993). Sociomedical researchers have contributed to this emphasis on behavioural explanations, with behaviours such as smoking becoming the main focus of many studies of health inequalities (MacIntyre 1986). These studies illustrate important methodological issues.

Ill-defined variables, confounding and multivariate analysis

The limitations of measures of socio-economic status based on the occupation of the male head of household have already been considered. These limitations are magnified when study results are subjected to various forms of multivariate analysis in order to identify a single variable, or group of variables, to account for most of the variance between social groups. Problems of confounding arise when the variables of interest are positively correlated to each other as well as to the outcome of interest. The use of ill-defined variables such as the Registrar General's Social Class may lead to the false conclusion that the effects of other variables such as smoking are 'independent' of social circumstances (Smith and Phillips 1992).

This effect is seen in studies of Sudden Infant Death Syndrome (SIDS). Every major case control and cohort study over the last twenty years has reported an association of poor social circumstances and SIDS. Recent studies, using occupational measures of socio-economic status, have concluded that parental, particularly maternal, smoking accounts for this difference and is one of the main determinants of SIDS (Gilbert *et al.* 1992; Mitchell *et al.* 1992). However, large US studies using income levels as the measure have shown that the effect of socio-economic status is modified but not eliminated by adjusting for maternal smoking (Kraus *et al.* 1988).

Bias in outcome measures and the confusion of biological and social variables

Just as poor definition of variables can lead to misinterpretation and inappropriate conclusions, so the introduction of bias into the outcome measure used in a study can have the same effect. Brooke *et al.* (1989) concluded that smoking was the most important explanatory variable for birth weight. However, they had used birth weight corrected for maternal height as the main outcome measure. As maternal height itself is positively correlated with socio-economic status, some of the effects were already controlled for in the main outcome measure. There is a tendency to classify some variables which are strongly influenced by social factors as 'biological'. Adult height and birth weight are two such variables. The effect of this misclassification is evident in a study of the determinants of height attained in mid-childhood (Gulliford *et al.* 1991) which concludes that the effects of socio-economic status on height are eliminated when adjustment is made for 'biological factors' such as parental height and the child's birth weight.

The biomedical model and the search for a single cause

Sociomedical researchers have tended to adopt the biomedical model of disease causation with its emphasis on the search for a single causal agent. This leads to the use of techniques such as multivariate analysis to identify the variable which has the strongest influence on the outcome of interest. The possibility of complex causal pathways (Rutter 1988) and cumulative effects of combinations of variables over time (Power *et al.* 1991) is excluded by these techniques. Rose (1992) suggests that the concept of 'proximal' and 'distal' causes better accounts for causal complexities than single cause explanations. In this model, socio-economic factors would act as distal causes of adverse health outcomes influencing more proximal causes such as diet and smoking.

The value of qualitative as well as quantitative data

Epidemiology is firmly based in quantitative research. As previously shown, quantitative research has made a major contribution to the identification and understanding of health inequalities. However, qualitative research also has an important place in the study of the privations of relative poverty and related health inequalities. Qualitative data from studies of poor families in the UK have shown, through the words of the poor themselves, the experience of living with relative poverty (Mack and Lansley 1984) and have provided invaluable insights into the reasons for poor nutrition (Land 1984) and smoking, especially amongst women who are caring for children

(Graham 1987). Qualitative techniques are particularly valuable for hypothesis generation. There is now a wide recognition of the value of both types of research and the value of combining both approaches in the study of social influences on health (Lewando-Hundt and Forman 1993). Neither form of research is exempt from the need for rigour in study design and data analysis.

STRATEGIES FOR REDUCING CHILD HEALTH INEQUALITIES

Drawing on the research findings discussed here, this section addresses the strategies which can be employed by health professionals and others working to reduce inequalities in child health. Health workers need to be fully informed of the magnitude and extent of health inequalities and committed to a non-victim-blaming approach which accepts other disciplines, and parents, as equal partners. The following discussion deals in detail with advocacy at national and local levels and strategies for protecting children from harm.

National strategies

In the UK, there is a particularly pressing need for health professionals to take political action on behalf of poor children and their families. Faced with a government which is reluctant to recognize the existence of poverty let alone its detrimental effects on health, child health workers must confront the political nature of the solutions required. The strategies for reaching *Health of the Nation* (Department of Health 1992) targets related to teenage pregnancy and childhood accidents, amongst others, focus on behaviour change and are invalidated by the failure to recognize the role of poverty and social disadvantage.

Health of the Nation does, however, encourage the development of 'healthy alliances' which can be used to challenge current orthodoxy. A recent example of this is the Public Health Alliance which has argued that smoking- and diet-related health promotion may be counter-productive if it fails to take account of the social context of behaviour (Laughlin and Black 1995). In concert with national groups such as the Child Poverty Action Group, the Maternity Alliance and National Children's Homes, health workers, individually and through their professional organizations, can bring research data to public attention and contribute to the development of alternative strategies for health gain.

Some countries have appointed Child Commissioners (in Norway and Sweden, known as Ombudsmen) whose task it is to represent the interests of children and monitor progress of the UN Convention on the Rights of the Child in their country. In the UK, there is a move to persuade politicians of the importance of such a post: an Office has been formed to promote this development which is supported by the British Association of Community Child Health. In New Zealand, the Commissioner has been able to bring the needs of poor Maori and Pacific Island children to public attention and influence policy related to the treatment of ethnic minority children.

Advocacy at national and local levels

If child health workers are to promote the health of children, they have to become not just providers of treatment and care during illness but advocates for children in order to protect them from forces beyond the control of the individual child and family which may damage their health and threaten their well-being. Advocacy for children is often limited to representing the child against its parents in child protection cases. The limitations of this approach are discussed in more detail later but advocacy can be a much broader concept. This can be illustrated using two specific examples: the prevention of childhood accidents and the provision of affordable and suitable housing for families with children.

Childhood accidents are now the commonest cause of child death beyond the age of one year. Road traffic accidents (RTAs) become an increasingly dominant cause of death as children get older. Accidents in the home, particularly fires, are more common in younger children (Woodroffe *et al.* 1993). Both RTAs and fatal accidents in the home show a strong social class gradient. Decontextualized health promotion strategies have concentrated on education of mothers. Recent evidence shows that health education alone is ineffective in reducing accidents (Sibert 1992). Strategies which modify the child's environment are needed in order to effectively prevent accidents (ibid.). Incidence of RTAs is increased by proximity to busy roads and strategies which separate residential areas from busy roads have proved effective (Towner *et al.* 1993). In the home, reliance on mobile gas and oil heaters, as well as structural problems and overcrowding, are associated with fatal accidents.

In the area of childhood accidents, advocacy which addresses the social context in which accidents occur might concentrate on the following issues:

- the evidence linking accidents to poor social conditions;
- the evidence linking residence in poor areas and proximity to heavy traffic with RTAs;
- the evidence demonstrating the relative effectiveness of environmental change over education strategies;
- the evidence linking home accidents to overcrowding, poor housing conditions and inappropriate forms of heating;
- lobbying national and local government to modify children's environments using traffic calming strategies and more long-term strategies which reduce reliance on the private car;
- forming healthy alliances with local and national lay and professional groups to influence transport and housing policy locally and nationally;
- promoting community participation and community diagnosis locally to identify the main sources of danger to their children from the perspective of community residents.

Waterston (1995) reports an initiative to prevent childhood accidents in Newcastle which utilizes some of these approaches to advocacy. Of particular interest is the use made of a survey by local parents which demonstrated a lack of safe crossing points on the children's route to school. These data were used by a multidisciplinary group to lobby for environmental change.

Affordable and suitable housing is almost uniformly recognized as essential for the well-being of families and children. Government policy over the last fifteen years has drastically reduced the stock of affordable housing and local authorities have been starved of capital for repairs with the result that there has been an increase in homes which are unfit for human habitation (Heath 1994). One result has been a sharp rise in homeless families who are accommodated at great expense in privately owned hotels and guest houses (ibid.). This accommodation is insanitary and overcrowded, with whole families often living in one room, using inadequate communal washing and toilet facilities. Health workers have contributed to the challenge to government housing policy (Heath 1994; Lowry 1991) and have advocated for children living in homeless accommodation (Parsons 1991).

Health workers have a particularly valuable role as advocates for housing improvements. They are in a position to provide the following, which can be used by inter-sectoral groups and those, such as Shelter, campaigning for the homeless:

• data on the health effects of inadequate housing and homelessness;
• data on the health effects of damp and mould;
• data on the health effects of overcrowding;
• data on the detrimental psychological effects of housing in-security;
• locally collected data on the health hazards of inadequately maintained dwellings;
• data collected through community participation related to the health effects of inadequate housing as perceived by the tenants themselves; and
• health workers can provide expertise to tenants' organizations in setting up surveys, carrying out interviews and data analysis.

The potential role of health workers in advocacy for children and their families struggling with the privations of life in poverty is considerable, as the examples considered here illustrate. Advocacy by health workers is not new: there is a long and honourable history of medical intervention on behalf of communities in order to promote the health of whole communities rather than just individuals within them.

Local strategies – for 'child protection'

Child protection has been dominated by the investigation of child abuse and neglect and the prosecution of perpetrators. In part, this domination is the result of a focus on 'family pathology' with little regard for the societal processes which create the climate and pressure in which abuse of children is likely to occur, so that child abuse is narrowly defined within the confines of the family. Gil (1970) has proposed a broader definition:

> any act of commission or omission by individuals, institutions, or society as a whole, and any conditions resulting from acts of inaction, which deprive children of equal rights and liberties, and/ or interfere with their optimal development, constitute abusive or neglectful acts or conditions.

Implicit in this definition is the responsibility of governments and societies for ensuring optimal conditions for child rearing which goes far beyond the narrow focus on dysfunctional families. Gil's definition helps to partially explain why children in economically disadvantaged homes seem to be more vulnerable to child abuse and neglect (Baldwin and Spencer 1993) and chimes with *The Lancet* editorial (1987) which stated 'child abuse thrives on poverty, social inequity, ignorance, racism and unemployment'. Social policies which increase family poverty and impede child rearing are likely to lead to an increase in child abuse and neglect along with other poverty-associated problems such as teenage pregnancy, school failure and truancy and drug abuse.

If child protection is viewed from this broad societal perspective, the current emphasis on individual risk strategies (Browne & Saqi 1988) in the prevention of child abuse and neglect, and in the protection of children from harm, has to change. Alternative community-wide strategies which foster social support and aim to reduce the overall risk for the whole population by reducing inequalities are likely to be more effective in the long term (Chamberlin 1988). Changes in national and international social policies will have the most powerful effect in creating a positive climate in which child rearing is enhanced rather than undermined. However, there is an important role for local health workers and local decision makers in promoting the development of local community-wide initiatives.

What are the key factors of such initiatives? The following is a composite of the features of successful community-wide strategies derived from Schorr (1988) and the Department of Social Policy, University of Newcastle (1991):

- comprehensive and intensive;
- needs-led flexible service rather than service-led;
- family and community oriented;
- easily accessible;
- staff with time and skills to develop relationships of respect and collaboration;
- social, emotional support and concrete help with specific requirements;
- participation and partnership with associated training and job opportunities; and
- full use of local resources.

Applying these principles in practice requires a long term strategy supported by all child-caring agencies locally and a shift away from crisis management as the main service response to child abuse. Child protection crises clearly have to be dealt with appropriately, but failure to institute effective preventive strategies offering support to parents struggling with child rearing in conditions of poverty will ensure an inexhaustible flow of crises which will overwhelm the child protection agencies. The 'stream of life' analogy presented by Chamberlin (1988) depicts the dilemma for the services: downstream all the agencies are trying to fish children out of the water whilst upstream, poverty and associated family dysfunction are causing children to fall into the stream. Community-wide strategies involve 'looking up stream', attempting to prevent children falling into the water by strengthening local support mechanisms which maximize the ability of families to rear their children.

Individual level strategies

Many health workers work mainly with individual children and families either in clinics or surgeries or in the family home. Even at this level, strategies for reducing inequalities can be employed. Poor families often experience poor services as a result of the operation of the 'inverse care law' (Tudor Hart 1971) – those most in need of services are least likely to receive them. The powerlessness associated with poverty and deprivation tends to lead to an unequal power relationship between client and health worker and class, cultural and language barriers can further impede communication. As a consequence, access to good child health care may be relatively difficult for poor families, whose children are more likely to need specialist as well as non-specialist child health services, and for families from minority communities, especially where English is not the first language.

Strategies at this level for reducing inequalities include ensuring access of poor families to high quality child health services. The basic principles are summarized below:

• accessible, flexible and relevant services 'free at the time of use';
• locally provided services of high quality minimizing the financial burden imposed by the need to travel to specialist services;
• health workers who respect parental skills and treat parents as genuine partners in the care of their children;
• health workers who recognize the special problems of caring for children in poverty and modify their case management and treatment regimes accordingly; and

- health workers who carry out non-discriminatory practice respecting cultural differences and recognizing the 'double jeopardy' faced by ethnic minority families.

CONCLUSIONS

This chapter has outlined the enhanced understanding of health inequalities in the fifteen years since the publication of the Black Report and the indications that inequalities are widening. It has discussed the issues of data interpretation which have influenced the causal debate and helped sustain the view that the health-related behaviour of the poor, and not poverty itself, is responsible for health inequalities. It has then considered strategies for health workers aimed at reducing health inequalities in a particularly vulnerable group – children.

The question must inevitably arise: with the understanding that we now have of health inequalities and the range of strategies available for reducing them, why are they continuing to widen? The first and most important response is the lack of political will, coupled with an ideological resistance to acceptance of the existence of relative poverty in society and its effects on health. Health is seen as an individual responsibility and the health and safety of children the main (sometimes the sole) responsibility of parents, regardless of their material circumstances. As noted, UK Government social policies, increasingly punitive to those families dependent on state benefits, are likely to be the underlying reason for widening child health inequalities.

The focus on health-related behaviour and individual responsibility for health has been strengthened and nurtured by some medical researchers. Health-related behaviours have been studied outside their social context and, where social context has been taken into account, the measures used have inadequately reflected the extent of material disadvantage. The search for a single causative agent has contributed to research conclusions and interpretations which serve to minimize the apparent influence of adverse social circumstances on health outcomes. Smoking has become the 'new scourge', the single most important health determinant, whilst poverty and material disadvantage, consistently shown to be equally powerful in their adverse effects, are either ignored or relegated to a minor role.

Further barriers to the reduction of health inequalities, though less significant, are the organizational changes and attitudes within the health services. The drive for increasing cost efficiency combined with the 'NHS reforms' is shifting resources from patient care to financial management and is tending towards a 'two-tier' service which will inevitably disadvantage the poor. Despite declarations of commitment to equity in service delivery, punitive and discriminatory attitudes to the poor and the disadvantaged remain a problem within the health services. Whilst the lack of political will to properly address health inequalities persists, it is likely that these attitudes will remain deeply embedded within the services.

For those health workers committed to health inequality, these barriers may seem insurmountable. However, the current orthodoxy of individual responsibility for health has been consistently challenged and is increasingly difficult to sustain in the face of the evidence summarized here. Further studies with material disadvantage as their focus are needed to deepen understanding of the processes by which health is affected. Decontextualized behavioural interpretations should be challenged as part of a continuing causal debate. Intervention studies using the principles previously outlined, are needed alongside collation and dissemination of the results of interventions which have been shown to work in the reduction of health inequalities. Use of some or all of the strategies outlined above will contribute to the pressure for political change and at the same time might even, if only marginally, improve the capacity of parents and families to protect and promote the well-being of their children.

REFERENCES

Baldwin, N. and Spencer, N.J. (1993) 'Deprivation and child abuse: implications for strategic planning', *Children and Society* 7(4): 357–75.

Brooke, O.G., Anderson, H.R., Bland, J.M., Peacock, J.L. and Stewart, C.M. (1989) 'The effects on birthweight of smoking, alcohol, caffeine, socioeconomic factors and psychosocial stress', *British Medical Journal* 298: 795–801.

Browne, K. and Saqi, S. (1988) 'Approaches to screening for child abuse and neglect', in Browne, K. Davis, C. and Stratton, P. (eds) *Early Prediction and Prevention of Child Abuse*, Chichester: Wiley.

Carstairs, V. and Morris, R. (1992) *Deprivation and Health in Scotland*, Aberdeen: Aberdeen University Press.

Chamberlin, R. (ed.) (1988) *Beyond Individual Risk Assessment: Community Wide Approaches to Promoting Health and Development of Families and Children*, Washington, DC: National Center for Education in Maternal and Child Health.

Cook, J., Pechevis, M. and Waterston, A. (1995) 'Community participation and community diagnosis', in Linstrom, B. and Spencer, N.J. (eds) *Social Paediatrics*, Oxford: Oxford University Press.

Cooper, J. (1991) 'Births outside marriage: recent trends and associated demographic and social changes', *Population Trends*, 63: 8–18.

Department of Health (1992) *The Health of the Nation: A Strategy for Health in England*, London: HMSO.

Department of Social Policy, University of Newcastle (1991) *The Walker Riverside Study: Report and Recommendations*, Newcastle: University of Newcastle Upon Tyne.

Dowler, E. and Calvert, C. (1995) *Nutrition and Diet in Lone-parent Families in London*, London: Family Policy Studies Centre.

Fox, A.J. and Shewry, M. (1988) 'New longitudinal insights into relationships between unemployment and mortality', *Stress Medicine* 4: 11–19.

Fox, A.J., Goldblatt, P.O. and Jones, D.R. (1985) 'Social class mortality differentials: artefact, selection or life circumstances?', *Journal of Epidemiology and Community Health* 39: 1–8.

Gil, D. (1970) *Violence against children*, MA: Harvard University Press.

Gilbert, R., Rudd, P., Berry, P.J., Fleming, P.J., Hall, E., White, D.G., Oreffo, V.O., James, P., Evans, J.A. (1992) 'Combined effects of infection and heavy wrapping on the risk of sudden unexpected infant death', *Archives of Disease in Childhood* 67: 171–7.

Gordon, R.R. (1986) 'Whatever happened to the Black Report?', *British Medical Journal* 293: 394.

Graham, H. (1987) 'Women's smoking and family health', *Social Science and Medicine* 25: 47–56.

Grimsley, M. and Bhat, A. (1986) 'Health', in Bhat, A. (ed.) *Britain's Black Population: A New Perspective* (2nd edition), Aldershot: Gower.

Gulliford, M., Chinn, S. and Rona, R. (1991) 'Social environment and height: England and Scotland, 1987 and 1988', *Archives of Diseases in Childhood* 66: 235–40.

Heath, I. (1994) 'The poor man at his gate', *British Medical Journal* 309: 1675–6.

Jarman, B. (1983) 'Identification of underprivileged areas', *British Medical Journal* 286: 1705–9.

Jones, I.G. and Cameron, D. (1984) 'Social class – an embarrassment to epidemiology', *Community Medicine* 6: 37–46.

Judge, K. and Benzeval, M. (1993) 'Health inequalities: new concerns about the children of single mothers', *British Medical Journal* 306: 678.

Kraus, J.F., Peterson, D.R., Standfast, S.J., van Belle, G. and Hoffman, H.J. (1988) 'The relationship of socio-economic status and sudden infant death syndrome: confounding or effect modification?', in Harper R.M. and Hoffman, H.J. (eds) *Sudden Infant Death Syndrome: Risk Factors and Basic Mechanisms*, New York: PMA Publishing Corporation.

Lancet (1987) 'Ill-treatment of children' (Editorial), 14 February.

Land, T. (1984) *Jam Tomorrow?* Manchester: Food Policy Unit, Manchester Polytechnic.

Laughlin, S. and Black, D. (1995) *Poverty and Health*, Birmingham: Public Health Alliance.

Le Fanu, J. (1993) *The Phantom Carnage*, London: Social Affairs Unit.

Lewando-Hundt, G. and Forman, M.R. (1993) 'Interfacing anthropology and epidemiology: the Bedouin Arab Infant Feeding Study', *Social Science and Medicine* 36: 957–64.

Lowry, S. (1991) *Housing and Health*, London: BMJ Publications.

MacIntyre, S. (1986) 'The patterning of health by social position in contemporary Britain: direction for sociological research', *Social Science and Medicine* 23: 393–415.

McCarron, P.G., Smith, G.D. and Womersley, J. (1994) 'Deprivation and mortality in Glasgow: increasing differentials from 1980 to 1990', *British Medical Journal* 309: 1481–2.

McLoone, P. and Boddy, F.A. (1994) 'Deprivation and mortality in Scotland, 1981 and 1991', *British Medical Journal*, 309: 1465–70.

Mack, J. and Lansley, S. (1984) *Poor Britain*, London: George Allen and Unwin.

Marmot, M.G. and Smith, G.D. (1989) 'Why are the Japanese living longer?', *British Medical Journal* 299: 1547 51.

Marmot, M.G., Shipley, M.J. and Rose, G. (1984) 'Inequalities in death: specific explanations of a general pattern', *The Lancet* 1: 1003–6.

Marmot, M.G., Smith, G.D., Stansfield, S., Patel, C., North, F., Head, J., White, I., Brunner, E. and Feeney, A. (1991) 'Health inequalities among British civil servants: the Whitehall II Study', *The Lancet* 337: 1387–93.

Martin, C.J., Platt, S.D. and Hunt, S.J. (1987) 'Housing conditions and ill health', *British Medical Journal* 294: 1125–7.

Mitchell, E.A., Taylor, B.J. and Ford, R.P. (1992) 'Four modifiable and other major risk factors for cot death: the New Zealand study', *Journal of Paediatrics and Child Health* 28 (Suppl. 1): S3–8.

National Children's Homes (1991) *Family Nutrition Survey*, London: NCH.

Oakley, A., Rigby, A.S. and Hickey, D. (1993) 'Women and children last? Class, health and the role of the maternal and child health services', *European Journal of Public Health* 3: 220–6.

—— (1994) 'Life stress, support and class inequality: explaining the health of women and children', *European Journal of Public Health* 4: 81–91.

Osborn, A.F. (1987) 'Assessing the socio-economic status of families', *Sociology* 21(3): 429–48.

Pamuk, E.R. (1988) 'Social class inequalities in infant mortality in England and Wales from 1921 to 1980', *European Journal of Population* 4: 1–21.

Parsons, L. (1991) 'Homeless families in Hackney', *Public Health* 105: 287–96.

Phillimore, P., Beattie, A. and Townsend, P. (1994) 'Widening inequalities in northern England', *British Medical Journal* 308: 1125–8.

Power, C., Manor, O. and Fox, A.J. (1991) *Health and Class: The Early Years*, London: Chapman and Hall.

Reading, R., Openshaw, S. and Jarvis, S.N. (1990) 'Measuring child health inequalities using aggregations of enumeration districts', *Journal of Public Health Medicine* 12: 160–7.

Rose, G. (1992) *The Strategy of Preventive Medicine*, Oxford: Oxford Medical Publications.

Royal College of Physicians of London (1994) *Homelessness and Ill Health*, London: Royal College of Physicians.

Rutter, M. (1988) 'Longitudinal data in the study of causal processes: some uses and pitfalls', in Rutter, M. (ed.) *Studies of Psychosocial Risk: The Power of Longitudinal Data*, Cambridge: Cambridge University Press.

Schorr, L. (1988) *Within our Reach: Breaking the Cycle of Disadvantage*, New York: Anchor Doubleday.

Sibert, J. (ed.) (1992) *Accidents and Emergencies in Childhood*, London: Royal College of Physicians.

Smith, G.D. and Phillips, A.N. (1992) 'Confounding in epidemiological studies: why "independent" effects may not be all they seem', *British Medical Journal* 305: 757–9.

Smith, G.D., Blane, D. and Bartley, M. (1994) 'Explanations of socio-economic differentials in mortality: evidence from Britain and elsewhere', *European Journal of Public Health* 4: 131–44.

Smith, G.D., Shipley, M.J. and Rose, G. (1990) 'The magnitude and causes of socio-economic differentials in mortality: further evidence from the Whitehall study', *Journal of Epidemiology and Community Health* 44: 265–70.

Spencer, N.J., Logan, S. and Lewis, M.A. (1993) 'Multiple admission and deprivation', *Archives of Disease in Childhood*, 68: 760–2.

Spencer, N.J., Logan, S., Scholey, S. and Gentle, S. (1995) 'Deprivation and bronchiolitis', *Archives of Disease in Childhood* (in press).

Towner, E., Dowswell, T. and Jarvis, S. (1993) *Reducing Childhood Accidents: The Effectiveness of Health Promotion Interventions – A Literature Review*, London: Health Education Authority.

Townsend, P. (1979) *Poverty in the United Kingdom*, Harmondsworth: Penguin.

Townsend, P. and Davidson, N. (1982) *Inequalities in Health: The Black Report*, Harmondsworth, Penguin.

Townsend, P., Phillimore, P. and Beattie, A. (1988) *Health and Deprivation: inequality and the north*, London: Croom Helm.

Tudor Hart, J. (1971) 'The inverse care law', *The Lancet* 27 February: 405–12.

United Nations Development Project (1994) *Human Development Report 1994*, New York: Oxford University Press.

Waterston, A. (1995) 'How can child health services help reduce health inequalities?', in Spencer, N.J. (ed.) *Progress in Community Child Health Volume I*, London: Churchill Livingstone.

Wilkinson, R.G. (1989) 'Class mortality differentials, income distribution and trends in poverty', *Journal of Social Policy* 18: 307–35.

Woodroffe, C., Glickman, M., Barker M. and Power, C. (1993) *Children, Teenagers and Health: The Key Data*, Milton Keynes: Open University Press.

World Health Organization (1995) *WHO Report 1995*, Geneva: World Health Organization.

Chapter 11

Researching women's health work

A study of the lifestyles of mothers on income support

Hilary Graham

INTRODUCTION

This chapter illustrates how sociological research can contribute to the development of critical perspectives on inequalities in health, with implications for both policy and practice. It does so by focusing on a study of mothers caring for children in households dependent on income support. Drawing on mothers' accounts of their daily lives, this study provides an example of how, through sociological research, a fine-grained understanding can be developed of the circumstances in which and routines through which women in low-income households work to promote the health of their families. Interweaving quantitative and qualitative data, the study uncovers the contradictory nature of this 'health work', with mothers' caring strategies resting on patterns of behaviour, like cigarette smoking, which place health at risk.

Patterns of behaviour seen as playing an aetiological role in health are referred to as 'lifestyles' in current health policies. They occupy the central place in the Government's health strategy, with changes in behaviour treated as holding the key to improvements in health (Department of Health 1992; Scottish Office 1992). 'Risk factor targets' have been set for changes in diet, cigarette smoking, including a separate target for smoking in pregnancy, and alcohol consumption. This emphasis on lifestyles and risk factors has been associated with an approach to health policy which downplays the significance of living conditions, both as a direct influence on health and as the context in which individuals seek to look after their health and the health of those they care for. However, the importance of understanding the everyday contexts of health-related behaviour and the contribution of sociology to this is the central concern of this chapter.

The study in question considers, specifically, the everyday contexts in which mothers work for health in households in receipt of income support. The 1994/5 scale rates provide £92.15 a week for a lone mother caring for two children under eleven and £113.05 for a mother bringing up two children under eleven within a cohabiting heterosexual relationship. One in five mothers in Britain with dependent children under the age of sixteen depend, in whole or in part, on this means-tested benefit: 1,500,000 mothers and 2,300,000 children under sixteen live in households receiving income support. In contrast, there are 600,000 men in households with children in receipt of income support (Department of Social Security 1994).

While claimant families represent a significant sub-group within the population, they have rarely been asked to provide an account of their health, lifestyles and living conditions. Instead, these dimensions have been studied separately, within two different fields of research concerned respectively with living standards and lifestyles; and obliquely, through measures of socio-economic status which shed only an indirect light on the context and patterns of health-related behaviour in claimant households. The following section outlines the research literature on living standards and lifestyles. This provides a backdrop to the discussion of the findings of the study of claimant mothers. The study formed part of a larger survey of mothers' experiences, carried out in the Midland counties of England in the early 1990s (Graham 1993). The survey's design meant that the majority of the mothers were White. It should be noted, therefore, that the study was not able to track the ways in which mothers' experiences of health-related behaviour were mediated by their ethnic identity and background and by their differential exposure to racism. Finally, the ways in which the study's findings illustrate the contribution that sociological research can make to policy and practice in the field of health are discussed.

RESEARCH ON LIVING STANDARDS AND LIFESTYLES

Living standards and lifestyles represent two distinct fields of research. Research concerned with living standards has recorded a rapid widening of inequalities in household income in Britain since 1979 (Goodman and Webb 1994). It is a process which has had a disproportionate impact on households with children. As a result, the proportion of families with incomes below the European Union decency threshold, defined as a household income less than

50 per cent of average household income, increased from 10 per cent in 1979 to 31 per cent in 1991 (Department of Social Security 1993). National statistics suggest that lone mother households have experienced a particularly sharp deterioration in their economic circumstances. As the numbers of lone mother households have increased, the proportion dependent on supplementary benefit/ income support has risen. In 1971, around one in three (37 per cent) of lone mothers were receiving supplementary benefit, the precursor of income support (Burghes 1993). Today, over 70 per cent of lone mothers live on income support. In contrast, less than one in ten lone fathers depend on this basic means-tested benefit (Bradshaw and Millar 1991).

In monitoring trends in household income and benefit status, research on living standards has documented the everyday lives of those at the bottom end of income distribution. Surveys have described the living standards and budgeting strategies of households on benefit, with households with children representing a particular focus of research (Bradshaw and Holmes 1989; Cohen et al. 1992; Kempson et al. 1994). Studies have indicated that the rates of income support paid to households with children are substantially below the level needed to secure a basic living standard, with the result that mothers are working for health in the face of unmet needs and unpaid (and often unpayable) bills (Kempson et al. 1994; Oldfield and Yu 1993). The struggle to keep children healthy and to avoid health-damaging behaviours is often vividly recorded in these surveys. However, their focus on living standards has typically precluded the systematic collection of data on individual health and health-related behaviour.

Instead, health-related behaviour and health have been studied within a separate seam of research. A series of large scale surveys have uncovered sharp socio-economic differences in women's lifestyles (Blaxter 1990; Office of Population Censuses and Surveys 1994; White et al. 1993). However, these surveys reveal little of the ways in which other dimensions of inequality are related to health-related behaviour (Graham 1995; Rudat 1994). In part, this is because minority groups, including minority ethnic groups, form only a relatively small proportion of nationally-representative samples. In part, it reflects the use of measures of social position which can obscure differences between women. For example, the classification of cohabitation status accords a privileged status to women's relationships with men. Cohabitation is defined exclusively in heterosexual terms, with women recorded either as living alone or as living with a male partner. As a result, the major lifestyle surveys are silent on the question of how the domestic lives of women living with women, in sexual and non-sexual relationships, affect their eating and smoking habits and their patterns of exercise and alcohol consumption. They are silent, too, on the broader question of if and how sexuality is expressed in lifestyles: on whether the meanings and patterns of diet, smoking and alcohol consumption are different for lesbians and straight women (Buenting 1993).

The major lifestyle surveys suggest that, at least for White heterosexual women, health-related behaviour tends to display a negative socio-economic gradient. Women in higher socio-economic groups are most likely to have lifestyles which match government targets while women in more disadvantaged circumstances are most likely to report lifestyles deviating from current medical advice. Thus, physical exercise is more common and more frequent among women at the top of the class ladder and women in higher socio-economic groups (SEGs) are more likely than women in lower SEGs to have fresh fruit every day and to avoid a daily diet of chips and fatty food (Cox 1987; White *et al.* 1993). Patterns of infant feeding mirror these differences in adult eating habits. White mothers in poorer circumstances are less likely to breast feed their babies at birth than mothers in more advantaged circumstances; a lower proportion also continue to breast feed their babies beyond six weeks (Figure 11.1). Low prevalence rates have also been uncovered in the limited range of studies of South Asian and African-Caribbean mothers caring for children in disadvantaged circumstances and inner-city communities (Costello *et al.* 1992; Department of Health 1994; Douglas 1989).

Socio-economic differences are etched deeply into the smoking habits of White mothers, with high rates of prevalence associated with low household income and low standards of living (Marsh and McKay 1994). As Figure 11.1 records, women with male partners in social class V have prevalence rates prior to pregnancy nearly three times higher than women in social class I.

Among women without a male partner to lock them into the class classification scheme, the majority (62 per cent) are smokers (Figure 11.1). In interpreting these figures, it should be noted that cigarette smoking has a strong ethnic identity, as a habit more common among White than African-Caribbean women and as a habit reported by only a small minority of South Asian women (Graham 1993; Marsh and McKay 1994; Rudat 1994).

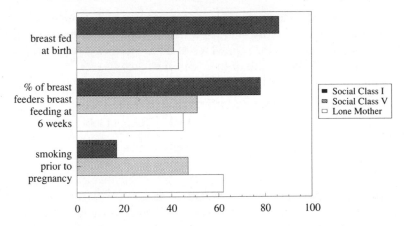

Figure 11.1 Patterns of infant feeding and cigarette smoking among mothers by social class (based on occupation of male partner), UK, 1990
Source White, Freeth and O'Brien (1992), Tables 2.3, 2.11 and 2.35

The drinking habits of White women display a different socio-economic profile. Alone among the major risk factors of female mortality, alcohol consumption is positively rather than negatively associated with socio-economic status and household income (Cox 1987). The highest proportion of women reporting that they were non-drinkers or drank less than one unit of alcohol a week is found among those in manual socio-economic groups (Office of Population Censuses and Surveys 1994; White *et al.* 1993). Conversely, it is those in the highest socio-economic groups who are most likely to drink more than the recommended sensible maximum per week (White *et al.* 1993). Among African-Caribbean and South Asian mothers, alcohol consumption rates are low (Douglas 1989; Department of Health 1994).

In charting socio-economic differences in health-related behaviour, surveys have relied primarily on the conventional (and problematic) measure of women's socio-economic position, based on the present or last occupation of male partners. The major alternative measures include housing tenure and car ownership, either on their own or as part of a composite measure of the living standards of women and children. To date, benefit status has not been included among these alternative measures and claimant households have typically comprised too small a sub-group to permit separate analyses of health, lifestyles and living conditions on income support.

The two sections below open up this important and complex area, describing findings from a study in which mothers on income support recorded the circumstances in which and the routines through which they worked for the health of their families.

INTRODUCING THE STUDY: THE SOCIAL AND MATERIAL CONTEXTS OF HEALTH-RELATED BEHAVIOUR

The study of mothers on income support is drawn from a larger survey of smoking patterns among lone and cohabiting mothers caring for babies of six months old (Graham 1993). The original survey was drawn from the records of two maternity hospitals and included White and African-Caribbean mothers in households where the head of household was either unemployed/ economically inactive or was employed in a manual occupation[1]. The majority (96 per cent) of the mothers identified themselves as White. Among the mothers who took part in the study, 242 were dependent, in whole or in part, on income support[2]. It is this group of mothers whose lives and lifestyles are the focus of this and the subsequent section.

The majority of the mothers on income support were under the age of twenty-five and were caring for children outside a cohabiting relationship with a male or female partner (Figures 11.2 and 11.3). Reflecting the younger age of their children, the proportion of single (never married) women is higher, and the proportion of separated and divorced women is lower, than in the general population of mothers on income support (Department of Social Security 1994).

Mothers' lives were structured around the daily routines of caring for young children. Only three mothers (1 per cent) reported that they were not with and caring for their baby on a full-time basis. A substantial minority (43 per cent) were caring for other pre-school children as well and, again, almost all were doing so on a full-time basis. Paid employment provided a break from childcare for less than one in ten (7 per cent) of the mothers. Mothers' domestic responsibilities extended beyond the routine provision of childcare to include the care of partners and children with acute and chronic illness or who experienced some form of impairment. Over a third (37 per cent) of the babies were reported to have a persistent cough and nearly half (47 per cent) had a persistent cold.

Indicators regarded as a sensitive measure of the living standards of white women, like housing tenure, suggest that the majority of the

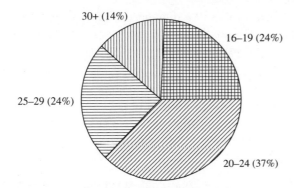

Figure 11.2 Age of mothers
(n = 242)

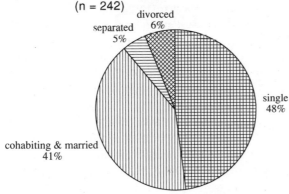

Figure 11.3 Cohabitation status of mothers
(n = 242)

mothers in the study were working for health without access to the material resources that most families take for granted. Nationally, 35 per cent of lone parent families and 76 per cent of two parent families are living in owner-occupied housing (OPCS 1991). Among the mothers in the study, only one in five (22 per cent) were in owner-occupied housing, with single women living with their parents making up a large proportion of this group. It should be noted that tenure provides a static measure of what was often an insecure and unstable housing situation, as the following accounts illustrate:

He (partner) had an accident at work and broke his wrist. He has had metal pins inserted. It happened about Christmas and he is still out of work. He shared his house with his sister and her husband, so when I became pregnant, there wasn't enough room and we had to find somewhere else to live. We thought we might have to go into bed and breakfast. We got this house about a week before she (daughter) was born. We were quite lucky really.

My husband's been sick and out of work for 18 months. He managed to get a job here but no accommodation. We're renting but it's expensive and the tenancy finishes in December and we'll be homeless if we can't find anywhere else. We've no money for our own home and we'll be back in bed and breakfast again.

(cohabiting mothers)

Other measures of environmental conditions suggest that mothers were caring for children in homes and neighbourhoods in which health hazards were a routine feature (Figure 11.4). Half of the mothers (51 per cent) reported that dangerous roads were a problem and the same proportion identified a lack of play space for children in the neighbourhood. Over half of the mothers also reported dogs as neighbourhood problems, with a third reporting litter and vandalism as problems. While their homes and neighbourhoods lacked the space in which their children could play, and play safely, few mothers had private transport to enable them to use facilities further away. Less than one in three mothers (30 per cent) lived in a household with a car or van. A significantly smaller proportion had access to this household resource. Only one in six (15 per cent) of

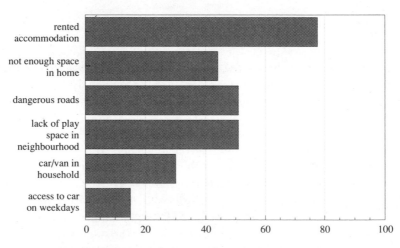

Figure 11.4 Housing and environmental problems
(n = 242)

the sample had access to a car/van during week days. While not a substitute for private transport, household ownership of a telephone can offset the effects of transport deprivation, providing mothers with a way of accessing health care routinely and in emergencies. However, the majority of the mothers (51 per cent) lived in accommodation without a telephone.

More subjective measures of living standards again suggest that the mothers were working for health in circumstances that denied them access to the material resources they needed. One of the questions asked mothers to assess how well their households were coping financially: to indicate whether their household was able to pay for all the things it needed, most of the things it needed, some of the things or hardly any of the things. Only one in five mothers (21 per cent) reported that their family was able to pay for all the necessities. The majority (57 per cent) noted that they were able to afford some or hardly any of the things they needed. In the struggle to make ends meet, items of personal expenditure, like clothes, were sacrificed to protect the living standards of their families. Thus, while the majority reported that they usually had enough money for food for their family (87 per cent) and for clothes for their children (70 per cent), only a minority of mothers (37 per cent) usually had enough money to pay for clothes for themselves.

> Bills are a problem. The problem is really when the money situation gets you really depressed, you might go out and buy something like some nice beefburgers and that makes it worse. We've got rent arrears of over £1,000 now. Every week the amount goes up.

> We've so many debts we don't know what to do.

> Fear of eviction is our biggest problem. It's still on-going. We have to go to court. If we can guarantee to pay they probably won't evict us. And the poll tax is a big problem. I received a letter saying they would take me to court as I hadn't paid it. I missed two payments.
>
> (cohabiting mothers)

The circumstances in which mothers were working for health were not only constrained by material shortages and insecurities. Mothers were also often labouring for health with limited health resources of their own. When asked to assess their health as excellent, good, fair or poor, only one in eight (12 per cent) rated it as excellent; four in ten (39 per cent) assessed their health as fair or poor. The national

Health and Lifestyle Survey provides comparative data on women aged 18 to 49 in households with high weekly incomes. In this group, 25 per cent rated their health as excellent and 16 per cent assessed it as fair to poor (Cox 1987).

Poor self-assessed health reflected the experience of a range of chronic health problems across the two weeks prior to the interview, like being constantly tired and having backache and headaches (Figure 11.5). It was also linked to the experience of long-term illness and physical impairment. One in four (26 per cent) reported long-standing illness or physical impairment, with asthma, impaired hearing and impaired movement (including arthritis and back and hip problems) figuring prominently in the mothers' replies.

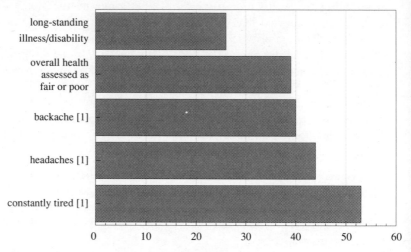

Figure 11.5 Patterns of mothers' health
(n = 242)
Note [1] within the two weeks prior to interview

The findings summarized in this section suggest that caring in the face of limited material resources and limited health resources provided the context within which health-related behaviours were sustained.

WORKING FOR HEALTH THROUGH HEALTH-DAMAGING BEHAVIOURS?

The routines of caring for children rest on behaviours which have become a focus of surveillance and intervention by health professionals, including infant feeding and cigarette smoking. The survey

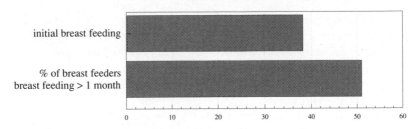

Figure 11.6 Patterns of breast feeding
        (n = 242)

confirmed the socio-economic patterning of these targeted behaviours. Reflecting the youthful age profile of the mothers, initial rates
of breast feeding were slightly below national prevalence rates for
mothers in social class V and lone mothers (see Figure 11.6). Among
mothers who initially breast fed, patterns of breast feeding at one
month are in line with national rates among mothers in the poorest
material circumstances (see Figure 11.6).

Smoking patterns are summarized in Table 11.1. The majority (61
per cent) of the mothers reported that they smoked one or more
cigarettes a day, with smokers clustered amongst those with relatively
high rates of cigarette consumption. Seventeen per cent of the smokers
reported that they smoked less than ten cigarettes a day, while more
than 40 per cent smoked twenty plus cigarettes a day. In the general
population of female smokers aged 16 to 34, the proportion of light
smokers is significantly higher (26 per cent) and the proportion
smoking more than twenty cigarettes a day is significantly lower (28

Table 11.1 Patterns of cigarette smoking
        (n = 242)

	%	(n)
Current smokers		
less than 10 a day	17	(23)
10–19 a day	43	(64)
20+ a day	41	(61)
Total current smokers	61	
Ex-regular smokers	13	(32)
Never or only occasionally	26	(62)
smoked a cigarette		
		(242)

per cent) (Office of Population Censuses and Surveys 1994).

High rates of prevalence and consumption were matched by low rates of never-smoking. Only one in four (26 per cent) of the mothers had never smoked: in the general population of women aged 16 to 34, the proportion is 54 per cent (Office of Population Censuses and Surveys 1994).

These smoking habits were sustained in the face of knowledge of the health risks of smoking. When asked if they thought that smoking was bad for people's health, 84 per cent of the mothers gave an unqualified yes. When those who qualified their answer in some way are included, the proportion rises to over 90 per cent. A lower proportion agreed that parental smoking was bad for the health of children. None the less, over 70 per cent gave an unqualified yes to the question; a proportion that rose to over 80 per cent when those who qualified their answer are included.

In contrast to their smoking behaviour, the drinking habits of mothers on income support were well within the limits prescribed by Government. Mothers noted how they cut down or gave up drinking in pregnancy and that, while they typically resumed their pre-pregnancy levels of drinking after birth, levels of consumption were generally low (Figure 11.7). The majority (62 per cent) of the mothers reported that they drank less than once a week. Only a small minority (3 per cent) reported drinking more than twice a week. These patterns stand in sharp contrast to those recorded by men in low-income households. National surveys suggest that nearly nine in ten (86 per cent) of men aged 18 to 39 in low-income households

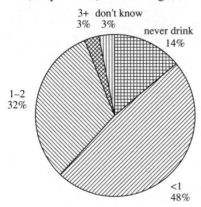

Figure 11.7 Patterns of alcohol consumption (times per week)
(n = 242)

have at least one drink a week. Nearly half report drinking moderately or heavily (Cox 1987).

Mothers' accounts of their smoking habits and drinking habits suggest that they formed part of a broader lifestyle fashioned out of the needs and constraints of caring for children on income support. While smoking cigarettes formed an integral part of this lifestyle, drinking alcohol was rarely part of the daily routine through which they tried to keep themselves and their families going. The difference in the meanings and contexts of these two patterns of behaviour is illustrated in the answers mothers gave to questions about when they were likely to smoke and to have an alcoholic drink.

When smokers were asked to identify any times and situations when they were very likely to smoke, the most common response was to describe structured and anticipated breaks from caring, when, if even for a few minutes, mothers could rest and refuel. For example, nearly half (47 per cent) of the smokers described routine breaks as times in which they were very likely to smoke; a similar proportion (44 per cent) also identified situations when they could relax. Nearly three in four (73 per cent) said they were very likely to smoke if they got a bit of time to themselves during the day. Their accounts suggest that, along with a cup of tea or coffee, smoking a cigarette gave access to personal space and adult time. These moments of relaxation could also mark out a social life beyond childcare, with cigarettes given and shared with partners, family and friends.

Times or situations mothers identified as ones in which they were very likely to want to smoke

In the evening, sometimes I can sit down. I'm always on the go but I grab one when I sit down.

In the afternoon when she has gone to bed and I can sit down for a few minutes.

When I have a cup of tea and when my mum comes over. When I'm drinking, I'm more inclined to smoke. When my husband smokes.

(cohabiting mothers)

When I get five minutes from the kids.

At night, when the kids are in bed, that's when I enjoy one. First thing in the morning, but mainly at night.

(lone mothers)

Cigarette smoking was not only a habit structured by the demands and routines of caring. It was a habit deeply woven into the *process* of caring, providing a way of managing and defusing stress. Childcare situations which mothers found stressful were the second most common context mothers described when asked the open-ended question about particular times and situations in which they were very likely to smoke. Answers to a follow-up question about smoking in the context of feeling on edge underlined the stress-management function of smoking. Nine in ten mothers (87 per cent) stated that they would be very likely to smoke if they were feeling on edge and needed to calm their nerves.

Times or situations mothers identified as ones in which they were very likely to smoke

I have noticed when something gets on top of me, I light a fag up and relax.

When the baby is screaming and won't shut up.

When my eldest son won't do as he's told and he answers me back.

When I'm making the tea. The two older ones come home from school, the baby's hungry and all four of them are hungry. They are all fighting and screaming and the dinner's cooking in the kitchen. I'm ready to blow up so I light a cigarette. It calms me down when I'm under so much stress.

(cohabiting mothers)

Smoking as a stress reduction strategy also figured prominently in the accounts that mothers gave for increases in consumption. For example, two mothers explained why they smoked more in pregnancy in the following way:

I more or less chain-smoked (in pregnancy). It was the other kids who caused the stress. I had three under 4 years and I was pregnant. It was just the pressures from the children. The worry about everything got me down. The kids, the house, the shopping. The worry about how I was going to cope with the new baby, having him so close to the others.

(cohabiting mother)

Coping with the babies. I wasn't able to cope with two of them on my own, with my husband away (in prison).

(lone mother)

As mothers' accounts suggest, cigarette smoking was a coping strategy to which mothers had direct and immediate access. It was experienced as a habit that helped mothers fulfil their domestic responsibilities, both on a routine basis and through the times of stress that punctuate the lives of women caring for young children. Its distinctive place in mothers' lives is underlined when accounts of smoking and drinking habits are compared. Very few mothers identified either the ordinary routines of childcare or coping with situations where their children were getting 'out of hand' as ones in which they would be very likely to drink. In contrast to the 73 per cent of smokers who said they would be very likely to have a cigarette if they got a bit of time to themselves during the day, only 1 per cent of the mothers who drank alcohol identified having time to themselves as a situation in which they were very likely to drink. A similarly small proportion (1 per cent) of the drinkers stated that they would be very likely to drink at times when their children were getting 'out of hand' and they were having difficulty coping. More drinkers (5 per cent) reported that they would be very likely to drink if they were feeling on edge and needed to calm their nerves. However, the proportion is still significantly below the 87 per cent of smokers who said that they would be very likely to smoke in this situation. Instead of being meshed into the routines and stresses of caring, having a drink appeared to be associated with times and locations where mothers were away from domestic responsibilities and from the domestic contexts in which they worked to meet them:

I go out occasionally with some friends up the street. It sounds awful going out but a group of us go to the pub about once in a couple of weeks. The men can go any time, any night, any Sunday.

When I was pregnant, I thought it was bad for the baby. I can have a drink now if I fancy it but I don't go out much. I don't drink in the house.

Before I had the baby, I was out every night of the week. Now I only go out once a week. I feel as if I want to drink to make my night. It makes me feel it's an evening off.

(cohabiting mothers)

CONCLUSIONS

For over a century, individual behaviour has been identified as a major cause of ill health and premature death in Britain. Maternal behaviour has figured particularly centrally in debates about the nation's health, with the unhealthy habits of mothers identified as the major cause of disease and death in childhood in the early decades of the century (Lewis 1980; Smith and Nicholson 1992).

As in the past, a lifestyle emphasis is strongly in evidence in today's health policies, with interventions framed in ways which separate individual behaviour from its social and material context. This chapter, however, has turned the spotlight on these contexts, using sociological research to explore the connections between living conditions and lifestyles. It has focused on a study of mothers on income support who were working for health at home.

The study suggests that the mothers' lives were structured by their 'health work' and are framed by their material circumstances. Health-related behaviours were woven into lives characterized by heavy caring responsibilities, poor health and limited access to material resources. Some behaviours, like alcohol consumption, occupied a marginal place in the routines that sustained mothers through each day. It was identified as a habit which, while health-damaging, was not essential to their survival. Cigarette smoking, in contrast, was seen as a deeply contradictory habit, which both undermined and promoted the welfare of their family. On the one hand, mothers recognized the health costs of smoking, for themselves and their children. On the other, they were aware of its pivotal place in the routines which kept them going, hour by hour and day by day. Cigarette smoking was experienced as a child-protective strategy, a resource which helped mothers cope with the demands of caring, both on a routine basis and through the periods of stress and crisis that punctuated their lives. For the mothers in this study, habits like smoking were experienced less as a lifestyle choice and more as a life compromise, taken, in full knowledge of the health risks, to protect the welfare of the family.

As a small scale study, caution must be exercised in generalizing from its findings. Associations between living conditions and life-styles do not demonstrate a direct causal pathway. The processes linking how mothers live and what mothers do are likely to be much more complex. None the less, the findings illustrate the contribution sociological research can make to policy and practice in the field of health. The experiences recorded by the mothers in the study remind those engaged in defining policy and developing practice of the complex interconnections between lifestyles and living conditions. The mothers' accounts bear testimony to the ways in which health-related behaviours are maintained within and against the constraining circumstances of everyday life. Their accounts raise questions about the separation of lifestyles and living conditions which underpins current health policy. They argue powerfully for a broadening of the national health strategy to include targets and interventions which act directly on the social and material contexts associated with health-damaging behaviour.

ACKNOWLEDGEMENTS

The survey of mothers was funded by the Department of Health. The views expressed, however, are those of the author alone.

NOTES

1 South Asian mothers were not included in the survey because of their low levels of smoking prevalence. The sampling criteria biased recruitment away from mothers and partners in non-manual occupations. As a result, the sample of claimant mothers may be more disadvantaged than the general population of mothers with young children dependent on income support. The high proportion of mothers in rented housing suggests that this is the case. However, low levels of owner-occupation also reflect the age profile of the sample and other measures, including household ownership of a car and a telephone, indicate living standards in line with national statistics for low-income households/households without an economically active head (Office of Population Censuses and Surveys 1991, 1994).

2 Recruitment to the original survey was stratified by smoking status, to yield a sample in which 50 per cent of the mothers were smokers. The smoking prevalence rate in the population from which the sample was drawn was 44 per cent. In order to ensure the representativeness of the sample of mothers on income support, smokers were randomly excluded from the original sample to produce a sample with an overall prevalence rate of 44 per cent prior to the identification of mothers on income support.

REFERENCES

Blaxter, M. (1990) *Health and Lifestyles*, London: Routledge.
Bradshaw, J. and Holmes, H. (1989) *Living on the Edge: A Study of the Living Standards of Families on Benefit in Tyne and Wear*, London: Child Poverty Action Group.
Bradshaw, J. and Millar, J. (1991) *Lone Parent Families in the UK*, DSS Research.
Buenting, J.A. (1993), 'Health lifestyles of lesbian and heterosexual women', in Noerager Stern, P. (ed.) *Lesbian Health: What Are the Issues?* London: Taylor and Francis.

Burghes, L. (1993) *One Parent Families: Policy Options for the 1990s*, York: Family Policy Studies Centre/Joseph Rowntree Foundation.

Cohen, R., Coxall, J., Craig, G. and Sadiq-Sangster, A. (1992) *Hardship Britain: Being Poor in the 1990s*, London: Child Poverty Action Group.

Costello, A., Shahjahan, M. and Wallace, B. (1992) 'Nutrition for Bangladeshi babies', *Community Outlook* 2 (4): 21–4.

Cox, B.D. (ed.) (1987) *The Health and Lifestyle Survey*, London: Health Promotion Research Trust.

Department of Health (1992) *The Health of the Nation: A Strategy for Health in England*, London: HMSO.

—— (1994) *Weaning and the Weaning Diet*, Report of the Working Group on the Weaning Diet of the Committee on Medical Aspects of Food Policy, London: HMSO.

Department of Social Security (1993) *Households Below Average Income 1979–1990/91: A Statistical Summary*, London: HMSO.

—— (1994) *Social Security Statistics 1994*, London: HMSO.

Douglas, J. (1989) 'Food type preferences and trends among Afro-Caribbeans in Britain', in Cruickshank, J.K. and Beevers, D.G. (eds) *Ethnic Factors in Health and Disease*, London: Wright.

Goodman, A. and Webb, S. (1994) *For Richer, for Poorer: The Changing Distribution of Income in the United Kingdom 1961–91*, London: Institute for Fiscal Studies.

Graham, H. (1993) *When Life's A Drag: Women, Smoking and Disadvantage*, London: HMSO.

—— (1995) 'Diversity, inequality and official data: some problems of method and measurement', *Health and Social Care in the Community* 3: 9–18.

Kempson, E., Bryson, A. and Rowlingson, K. (1994) *Hard Times? How Poor Families Make Ends Meet*, London: Policy Studies Institute.

Lewis, J. (1980) *The Politics of Motherhood: Child and Maternal Welfare*, London: Croom Helm.

Marsh, A. and McKay, S. (1994) *Poor Smokers*, London: Policy Studies Institute.

Office of Population Censuses and Surveys (1991) *1989 General Household Survey*, London: HMSO.

—— (1994) *1992 General Household Survey*, London: HMSO.

Oldfield, N. and Yu, A.C.S. (1993) *The Cost of a Child: Living Standards for the 1990s*, London: Child Poverty Action Group.

Rudat, K. (1994) *Health and Lifestyles: Black and Minority Ethnic Groups in England*, London: Health Education Authority.

Scottish Office (1992) *Scotland's Health: A Challenge to Us All*, Edinburgh: HMSO.

Smith, D.F. and Nicholson, M. (1992) 'Poverty and ill health: controversies past and present', *Proceedings of the Royal College of Physicians, Edinburgh* 22: 190–9.

White, A., Freeth, S., and O'Brien, M. (1992) *Infant Feeding 1990*, London: HMSO.

White, A., Nicholas, G., Foster, K., Browne, F. and Carey, S. (1993) *Health Survey for England*, London: HMSO.

Chapter 12

Developing with Black and minority ethnic communities, health promotion strategies which address social inequalities

Jenny Douglas

INTRODUCTION

This chapter aims to explore the role of health promotion in opposing the impact of racism and racial discrimination on the health of Black and minority ethnic communities in the UK.[1] First, it examines some of the constraints and dilemmas health promotion faces at present, particularly in relation to addressing inequality in these communities. Second, it considers information currently available on the health of Black communities, concentrating on differential health experience and health status in relation to mortality and morbidity and the way in which work on health issues has tended to be conceptualized within minority ethnic communities.

The chapter then discusses lessons emerging from health promotion strategies which do aim to tackle inequality in Black and minority ethnic communities, drawing upon work that has been developed in Sandwell and focusing on the Smethwick Heart Action Research Project. This project has set out to document the health experience of these communities, opening up the links between poverty, racism and health and highlighting gaps in service provision. The project has also encouraged the participation of voluntary organizations and community groups in determining appropriate methods for health promotion. However, its initiatives too emerge as subject to current constraints on health promotion.

THE ROLE OF HEALTH PROMOTION

Health promotion is a relatively recent phenomenon, whose concepts and associated strategies and approaches developed out of health education (Tones 1983). One of the earliest attempts at defining the field of health promotion in its own right was produced by Lalonde in 1975 in *A New Perspective on the Health of Canadians*. The aim of this report was to move away from a narrow 'medical model' view of health and to define health promotion as an activity which aimed to take account of both structural and lifestyle factors in initiatives designed to foster health. The World Health Organization (WHO) Alma Ata Declaration in 1977 committed all member countries to the principles of 'Health for All', the key elements of which are

- reducing inequalities in health and ensuring equity in health;
- increasing community involvement and participation and promoting community development;
- encouraging inter-sectoral/multi-sectoral collaboration and alliances;
- developing international co-operation and learning from good practice;
- emphasizing and promoting primary health care.

(World Health Organization 1978)

In keeping with this approach WHO defines health promotion as a process of enabling people to increase control over, and to improve their health (World Health Organization 1984; World Health Organization undated). These developing ideas about health promotion have resulted in the identification of five key priority areas: building healthy public policy, creating supportive environments, strengthening community action, developing personal skills and reorienting health services (World Health Organization 1986).

However, the current national strategy for health promotion in Britain – *The Health of the Nation* (Department of Health 1992) – adheres to a narrower approach. It places emphasis on changing individual behaviour as a key strategy to improve health (Adams 1994), concentrating on the idea that people need information to help them make the right choices and that reliable health education in its widest sense is essential for this. Thus many health promotion programmes are now predicated on the notion of enabling people – individuals and communities – to make 'healthier' choices. But this notion assumes that individuals have control over their lives and their health, in order to be able to make those choices. It is clear that for many people the social, economic and political factors which impinge upon their health lie far beyond their immediate control. The *Health of the Nation* strategy does not, for example, acknowledge or refer to the impact of relative poverty on health despite the number of reports emphasizing the significance of this (Benzeval and Judge 1995; Townsend *et al.* 1992; Whitehead 1992) and the association between inequality and health (Wilkinson 1992). As Adams (1994) argues, health promotion is now in crisis, with people practising health promotion being expected to focus on quite narrow issues to the detriment of work on the underlying causes of ill health. Health promotion workers need to bring together economic, social and environmental agendas linked to health and these should be the framework for health promotion at a local level.

More specifically, current theories and concepts of health promotion do not tend to focus on the contemporary realities of racial discrimination and racial oppression. Where anti-oppressive practice has been developed, this has not arisen out of prevailing health promotion theories, but has tended to represent the attempt of individual practitioners to develop health promotion programmes and strategies that seek to address oppression (Douglas 1995a). The predominant approach adopted within health promotion campaigns and strategies is a multicultural one which concentrates on the particular cultures of Black and minority ethnic communities. It attempts to develop health promotion programmes and resources targeted at specific Black and minority ethnic communities, but without acknowledging the association between material inequality and ill health in the communities concerned. It also fails to move beyond a focus on the biological causes of ill health and their treatment by medical intervention (Douglas 1995b). In these respects it echoes some of the dominant assumptions informing medical research and health initiatives more generally within Black and minority ethnic communities. These are discussed next.

THE HEALTH OF BLACK AND MINORITY ETHNIC COMMUNITIES

An emphasis on the relative incidence of ill health

There is now a diverse and growing literature on the health of Black and minority ethnic communities. This has been reviewed by Smaje (1995), who demonstrates its continued emphasis on a biomedical model, with a focus on illness and diseases affecting the afore-mentioned communities. He argues that epidemiological work on mortality and morbidity has tended to concentrate on two approaches in examining the health of particular ethnic groups. The first approach is to outline the frequency of disease within each ethnic group by looking at prevalence or incidence of particular diseases or conditions, whilst the second approach is concerned with difference between ethnic groups. This is measured by relative risk or standardized mortality ratios which indicate the degree of difference between such groups. Bhopal (1988) has argued that the medical literature on the health of Black and minority ethnic communities has been inappropriately dominated by studies of relative risk. There has been an over-emphasis on diseases with high relative risk among Black and minority ethnic populations as compared to the White population, considered as the norm. Such an approach reinforces an emphasis on diseases such as tuberculosis and thalassaemia, where the diseases in question are ones where occurrence may reflect geographical or genetic aetiology. This is rather than concentrating on illnesses and conditions which affect larger populations of Black and minority ethnic people, such as coronary heart disease, where there may be explanations that relate to racially disadvantaged economic and social conditions.

In relation to morbidity, there is also little literature on the subjective experiences Black and minority ethnic communities have in relation to illness or disability. Where there is information this is usually not available at a national level, but is based upon small local studies of chronic illness or self-reported morbidity (Pilgrim *et al.* 1993; Thompson *et al.* 1994). Moreover, most health and lifestyle surveys have also been based on predominantly White populations (Blaxter 1990), and there is little national data available on the health and lifestyles of Black and minority ethnic communities. To counteract this tendency the Health Education Authority recently commissioned MORI's Health Research Unit to carry out a programme of health and lifestyle research on its behalf (Rudat 1994). This survey demonstrated that there were significant differences between White and other ethnic groups in relation to health status and perceptions of health. At least twice as many African Caribbean, Indian, Pakistani and Bangladeshi respondents defined their health status as poor when compared with White respondents.

The health agenda within Black and minority ethnic communities

The health agenda coming from Black communities has also tended to focus on the incidence of freedom from disease and on securing appropriate medical intervention. These have been important issues in their own right. For Black communities, community initiatives or campaigns around health issues have arisen out of the link between racial discrimination and the lack of appropriate service provision as in the case of sickle cell anaemia, thalassaemia, coronary heart disease, diabetes, hypertension and circumcision (Douglas 1991) or misdiagnosis based upon racial and cultural stereotypes, as in the case of mental illness (Wilson 1993). However, there has been little attention to the association between poverty, racism and ill health. Moreover, the women's health movement has not focused on the needs of Black and ethnic minorities and on the possible associations between sexism, relative poverty, racism and ill health (Douglas 1992). Little attention has also been focused on learning why some minority ethnic groups experience lower levels of certain diagnoses than the majority White population (Blakemore and Boneham 1993).

The association between socio-economic conditions and the health of Black and minority ethnic communities

A number of studies indicate that Black and minority ethnic communities experience relative disadvantage in relation to poverty and discrimination. With the exception of Chinese communities and East African Indians, unemployment rates for minority ethnic communities are much higher than for the White population (Amin and Oppenheim 1992; Brown 1984; Jones 1993). Rates of long-term unemployment are greater for most minority ethnic groups and the differential between minority ethnic groups and White communities has widened during the 1980s and is wider amongst young people (Amin and Oppenheim 1992; Jones 1993). Black people are also employed disproportionately in low-paid occupations and in poor working conditions such as night work and shift work (Brown 1984). A greater proportion of Black people are employed as home workers as compared to White people. Housing tenure shows ethnic patterns (Jones 1993), with African-Carribean and Bangladeshi people more likely to be living in rented council accommodation compared to the White population. Although people from Indian and Pakistani communities tend to be owner-occupiers, there is evidence that such ownership may still reflect occupancy of less expensive housing stock (Rudat 1994).

An association between low socio-economic status and poor health in the White population has been demonstrated, as referred to earlier, with poor health shown to be associated with poverty, unemployment, poor housing and poor working conditions. We have also discussed an association between minority ethnic status and disadvantage. Therefore material disadvantage associated with racism is a plausible explanation for poor health amongst Black and minority ethnic groups. However, there has been little research on the direct impact of the material disadvantage associated with racism upon the health experience of these groups. Some research has also suggested that poor health and ethnic differences in disease prevalence can be explained by other factors such as the geographical distribution of Black and minority ethnic populations who reside primarily in inner-cities (McIntyre 1986, Williams *et al.* 1994).

At most, the evidence on the effect of material disadvantage on Black and minority ethnic communities' health in the United Kingdom is therefore circumstantial. But what follows from this is that at the least, this issue should be a focus for further research and should be taken into account as a possibly significant factor in health promotion projects.

HEALTH PROMOTION, DISADVANTAGE AND ILL HEALTH

The aims of the Sandwell Unit

The preceding discussion demonstrates that there is a need for health promotion work to tackle the association between racism, disadvantage and ill health but that there are formidable conceptual and organizational barriers to doing so, in addition to the complexity of the task. At Sandwell the focus is on addressing racism and racial discrimination within a wider context of anti-discriminatory practice. This perspective not only informs the health promotion programmes that are developed in the locality, but also seeks to inform the employment practice of the Health Promotion Unit. The Unit actively seeks to address oppression in relation to class, gender, 'race', disability and sexuality. However, as well as there being few models of health promotion that emphasize the need to oppose and challenge racism and racial disadvantage, there is also little discussion of ways of addressing oppression in its wider forms. For example, the emphasis recently on developing specific HIV/AIDS campaigns and health promotion programmes focusing specifically on sexual health has meant that often health promotion work on gay or lesbian health needs has had a narrow focus on sexual behaviour. The starting point for health promotion initiatives in Sandwell has been to recognize and acknowledge that social, economic, environmental, political and cultural factors affect health. Thus health promotion strategies and programmes must be directed at community empowerment, i.e., raising awareness among local people of the factors that affect health, and at changing public policy: the policies of health authorities and trusts, local authorities and central government.

In adhering to such aims health promotion programmes must not, however, slip back into a didactic approach but must connect with people's own concerns. In keeping with this, another key principle of work in Sandwell has been to ensure that local people are involved in setting local priorities and in developing appropriate, acceptable and sustainable health promotion initiatives which acknowledge, respect and value the contribution of local people, community workers and health workers. I have outlined in an earlier section that for Black people, the focus is often on medical intervention and campaigning for appropriate services. Therefore, it has been important to address issues that Black and minority ethnic communities themselves raise: such as the incidence of coronary heart disease, diabetes, sickle cell anaemia, thalassaemia and infant mortality; provision for circumcision, the provision of interpreting services and appropriate hospital and community health services, as these have been immediate health concerns. One element of the health promotion programme which illustrates key issues and lessons related to this approach is the Smethwick Heart Action Research Project.

INTRODUCTION TO THE SMETHWICK HEART ACTION RESEARCH PROJECT (SHARP)

The Smethwick Heart Action Research Project was located within the framework of Healthy Sandwell 2000 and was a collaborative project between a number of agencies – the health authority, family health services authority, Health Education Authority – but located within the Sandwell Health Promotion Unit. SHARP grew from the community-based approach of Sandwell Health Promotion Unit, supported by and building upon networks and resources which had already been established. As a piece of action research in line with Torkington's discussion of similar work in Liverpool (1991), the project was designed to provide data which could reflect issues of relevance for local communities and hence influence local policies which aimed to improve the health of the population in general and Black and minority ethnic communities in particular.

The project was funded by the Health Education Council for three years from April 1991; its aims were to identify risk factors for Black and minority ethnic communities in Smethwick in relation to coronary heart disease and stroke. Although the focus was pre-determined as being on the incidence of disease, we sought to examine social, economic and political factors which might affect the health of these communities in Smethwick and to identify the priorities that members of Black communities worked to in terms of improving health.

The project's research approach

As discussed earlier, there is limited research on the health and lifestyle of Black and minority ethnic communities in the UK; but in order to start to address inequalities it is necessary to have some documentation of the experiences of these communities, not only in relation to longstanding illness and disability, but also in terms of the direct and indirect experiences of racism and racial discrimination in relation to health and social services. Some researchers have attempted to do this. Pilgrim et al. (1993), for example, highlight the experiences of Black and minority ethnic communities in Bristol, where respondents felt that they experienced racial discrimination in ways which undermined their health.

The project was also committed to developing appropriate research methodologies for ascertaining the health and social needs of Black and minority ethnic communities in Smethwick. Thus, an attempt to build in an anti-racist perspective and to involve local Black and minority ethnic communities was integral to the development of research questions, research protocol, research design and methodology. The methodology for the Smethwick Heart Action Research Project is discussed in detail in a number of documents (Thompson, Douglas and McKee 1994; Thompson, Malik, Douglas and McKee 1994). Here it is important to note the following points: the project steering group was composed of a group of people with research skills and from a range of ethnic backgrounds, to help to ensure that Black perspectives were built into the research project at the onset. In addition, before the project commenced, a range of community organizations and voluntary organizations were contacted and a consultation meeting held in conjunction with a local Asian Resource Centre, to outline the parameters of the project and to seek the views of local Black and minority ethnic people about what should be the aims and scope of the project. This was to ensure that areas identified for research and for future health promotion action were in accord with the needs local people identified.

Three hundred individuals from African Caribbean, Bangladeshi, Indian, Pakistani and White communities in Smethwick were interviewed using a structured questionnaire. A quota sampling method was used so that equal numbers of individuals from the five ethnic groups were interviewed and there were equal numbers of men and women. Interviews were conducted by interviewers matched for ethnicity and language to help to ensure that authentic information was collected.

To complement the research findings and provide an easily accessible database which was readily accessible to local individuals and community groups, a community health profile was developed alongside the SHARP survey. Drawing in part on census returns, historical, demographic and environmental information was assembled on the locality, together with a directory of community resources such as religious organizations, leisure services and mother and baby groups (Henry et al. 1993).

Key findings

Detailed discussion of further findings is provided elsewhere (Thompson, Douglas and McKee 1994; Thompson et al. 1994). Overall, on the basis of self-report evidence in this study, Bangladeshi communities and Pakistani communities appear to experience greater relative poverty, with higher rates of unemployment and more worries about money. However, the data outlines a complex picture of the differences between ethnic groups in terms of perception of health, social disadvantage, experiences of racial discrimination, money worries and debt, and communication. Focusing in on the first three issues:

Perception of Health

The findings demonstrated clear differences between Black and minority ethnic groups and White groups in relation to perceptions of health status. When asked, 'How healthy do you feel?' at least 17/60 in each of the Black and minority ethnic groups, compared with only 5/60 in the White group, answered 'not healthy' or 'not healthy at all'. The numbers were greatest for Pakistani (23/60) and Bangladeshi (22/60) respondents (Thompson, Douglas, McKee 1994).

Social Disadvantage

With the exception of Indian respondents, respondents from other minority groups were, for example, consistently less likely to be car owners than White respondents. When asked about housing problems, for example, damp, condensation or mould, major repairs outstanding or problems maintaining adequate heating – 63 per cent of people from the Bangladeshi group compared to 40 per cent of people from the Pakistani group, 28 per cent of African Caribbeans and Whites and 15 per cent of Indians stated they had housing problems.

Racial Discrimination

Nine per cent of the Black and minority ethnic sample reported racial discrimination and attacks as being a problem in the locality. This result can be compared to Pilgrim *et al.*'s Bristol survey (1993) where 11 per cent of people had experienced racial insults in the streets. Fifteen per cent of the Black and minority ethnic sample also felt that racism had affected their access to health services.

These findings illustrate the difficulty, but also the importance of beginning to disentangle such issues and their possible bearing on health, by obtaining information from different minority ethnic groups and not simply contrasting the position of members of one minority ethnic group and the White population.

The survey also sought to explore possible gender differences in health experience. The data relating to this is still being analysed. However, for example, in relation to experience of signs of stress, indications of women being at some disadvantage have emerged, although such differences require some qualification, and there is evidence of the interaction of gender and ethnic identity. Respondents were interviewed about feeling angry or irritable, feeling tired and finding it hard to relax. Forty three per cent of women in the survey as compared to 25 per cent of men said that they often felt angry or irritable with those around them. However, this was more frequently experienced by African-Caribbean and White women than other groups. In the African-Caribbean and White groups, just over half the women interviewed said that they often felt angry or irritable. At least one third of women in each group agreed that they felt very tired and had little energy. Overall, 47 per cent of women compared with 33 per cent of men experienced this. Forty-one per cent of women overall and 31 per cent of men found it very hard to relax and unwind.

Following on from such responses, the people interviewed highlighted a range of initiatives which they felt would improve their health. Across both White and minority ethnic groups, these related not only to initiatives they could take as private individuals such as to take more exercise, eat more healthily and to take steps to be happier in close relationships. They also concerned initiatives which drew on social policy measures such as provision of employment, good working conditions, a good standard of housing, a good education, to be reunited with family members abroad who were separated by immigration legislation and to live in a safe, clean environment. Thus the survey uncovered the way in which initiatives identified by Black and minority ethnic communities as having the potential to improve their health moved away from a 'medical model' focus. The respondents identified environmental, economic, political and cultural factors as affecting their health and their comments were much more aligned to the 'Health for All' model of health (World Health Organization 1978) cited earlier.

In the context of one-to-one interviews, the SHARP project therefore picked up a much broader definition of health than that which earlier research or community consultations had featured (Douglas 1991). The reason for this may be that, previously, community consultations had often focused upon Black health issues which had already become politicized: sickle cell disease and thalassaemia, mental health and circumcision (ibid.). In responding to health concerns, health promotion workers must, however, be able to address both this narrower health agenda, and the wider health agenda revealed by our survey. Unless the lack of health service provision is addressed, community support and trust will not be harnessed in order to tackle the much bigger issues of poverty, poor housing, material and racial disadvantage.

Further outcomes of the project

The project broke new ground in establishing that health promotion workers and respondents from Black and ethnic minority communities shared concerns about the impact of unequal social conditions on health, and about the importance of addressing these issues. This has also provided a focus for subsequent practice. A series of health promotion initiatives has arisen out of the needs identified by Black and minority ethnic communities during the survey. These have involved Black and minority ethnic communities in their planning, implementation and evaluation and have endeavoured to tackle aspects of disadvantage and discrimination injurious to health. Four are presented in detail here:

Interpreting services

In relation to communication, the survey showed that a third of the Bangladeshi group was literate only in Bengali, approximately one-quarter of the Pakistani group was literate only in Urdu and almost a quarter of the Indian group were literate only in Punjabi. Thus the research demonstrated that in Smethwick almost a quarter to a third of Asian communities were literate only in their first language, hence also demonstrating the need for appropriate translation and interpreting services. These research findings on language and experiences of discrimination were fed directly into the health services' commissioning machinery and led to a further investigation of interpreting services and a review of the overall provision of multilingual information.

SHARP Training Project

This project aimed to develop skills and confidence among Black and minority ethnic people/community workers in organizing health promotion activities. One of the reasons for this initiative was that, during community consultations, Black and minority ethnic people said that they felt that health promotion activities did not target Black and minority ethnic communities and that there should be more health promotion activities organized within temples, Gurdwaras and community centres used by Black and ethnic minority groups.

A training course was developed on 'Organizing groups and

activities in the Community'. This course was accredited by the Black Country Access Federation. Eight people attended the course which provided:

* personal development in a supportive environment;
* demystification of 'health promotion' – enabling local people/ community workers to develop skills in health promotion;
* networking between local community workers;
* development of health provision and awareness of health issues in organizations/community groups.

Promoting Asian foods as healthy

When asked about their health, one of the reasons people from Black and minority ethnic communities cited for feeling less healthy than the indigenous White population was their diet. Asian respondents described themselves as 'not eating right foods' and Asian foods as 'rich in fat', i.e., they appeared to view their food as unhealthy. Among respondents and workers, there was also the impression that White health professionals lacked awareness of Asian and African Caribbean foods and therefore perpetuated racist stereotypes about unhealthy Asian and Caribbean food customs/practices.

The Community Action Steering Group for this project therefore felt that it was important to:

* challenge myths about Asian foods with local Asian women and health professionals;
* promote healthy eating with Asian foods.

The health promotion project therefore organized one-day seminars on Food and Diet in a multiracial society, aimed at health visitors, community workers and local authority workers, to look at broader aspects of healthy eating in a multiracial society and also at the difficulties of affording food in low-income families. This second focal point was a crucial matter of concern as, in the SHARP survey, 24 per cent of respondents overall had said affording food was sometimes, often, or very difficult. Bangladeshi groups (41 per cent) and White groups (31 per cent) stressed that affording food was difficult. Twenty-five per cent of African Caribbeans and 10 per cent of Indian and Pakistani groups also said affording food was difficult.

Cookery demonstrations were also organized at a local community centre by Asian Community Liaison Officers from the FHSA (Family Health Services Authority) who had been involved with the

SHARP project. The aim of the workshops was to raise awareness of healthy eating with Asian foods and to demonstrate methods of reducing the fat content of meals. The demonstrations also included the use of cheaper, English vegetables, for example, leeks and potatoes, in place of more expensive traditional Asian vegetables, while still using Asian methods.

Sustaining health promotion initiatives

One of the shortcomings of SHARP was that it was a short-term funded project and hence it was important to try to ensure that its activities and initiatives were sustainable, by building upon networks that had been created. In achieving sustainability it is important to work with existing structures and representatives and workers within existing localities. It is important to involve established organizations including youth and community services, voluntary agencies, places of worship, community centres, local shops and health centres in any health promotion initiatives. For example, the SHARP survey had indicated low rates of physical/leisure activity among the Muslim population and 'Asian' women. Bangladeshi and Pakistani groups participated least in leisure exercise, as there were few facilities which catered for the needs and wishes of these communities. Facilities clearly needed to become more generally user-friendly, providing privacy for women, women instructors and information in Asian languages. Two key issues that emerged as the availability of appropriate facilities was explored were: the lack of local authority leisure services' provision of sessions for women-only in Smethwick; and stereotypical views among White professionals and organizations about Asian women, such as: religious beliefs prohibited them from participation in physical activity.

Consequently, two options were explored and developed in conjunction with the leisure department: providing Bhangra aerobics sessions at a community centre and providing swimming sessions for Asian women in Smethwick. The local authority Leisure Services Department employed a female Asian Sports Development Officer who worked with the SHARP team to develop the initiatives described above and these were then continued by the Leisure Services Department after initial piloting and evaluation through the SHARP project.

Democratic, participatory forms of evaluation also need to be built into all health promotion programmes and initiatives, which involve local people and communities not only in identifying their own ideal objectives but in reviewing the outcomes. Each health promotion initiative developed as part of the Smethwick Heart Action Research Project had a community action steering group with members drawn from local community groups and voluntary organizations. These consulted with local people and organizations not only before the development of health promotion programmes – identifying the possible options and in implementing the health promotion pro-grammes – but also in evaluating their success (Malik, Thompson, Douglas and McKee 1994).

CONCLUSION

The Smethwick Heart Action Research Project has demonstrated that health promotion can start to identify key issues and concerns for local people trying to maintain and improve health against a backcloth of social disadvantage, notably, for Black and minority ethnic communities, against racism and racial discrimination. The findings from SHARP show that Black and minority ethnic com-munities are in fact aware of the social, economic and environmental factors influencing their health. What is more difficult is to develop health promotion programmes which address such concerns, once they have been identified. This project, within the limitations of its funding, tried to achieve small changes in policies within health and local authorities and to empower local communities to develop health promotion programmes which focused not only on lifestyle approaches to heart health but which acknowledged the impact of material factors.

SHARP also demonstrates that it is possible to make progress on the self-direction of health promotion initiatives by members of the local community, which address these issues.

However, in other respects, the experience of SHARP makes sobering reading. More sophisticated methods need to be developed to assess the health needs of black and minority communities, which reflect diversity in terms of ethnicity, 'race', culture, class, gender and disadvantage. Nationally, the remit of current health promotion practice is constrained by the *Health of the Nation* strategy, which does not offer an incentive to move beyond a narrow focus on individual behaviour change as affecting the incidence of disease.

It is important for health promotion to develop methodologies and practices which recognize the social, economic and environmental factors affecting health. In doing so, as SHARP's experience demonstrates, there is a need for health promotion to develop strategies to work with other organizations which are better placed to effect changes in policy to improve health. Local respondents to SHARP's survey clarified, for example, that substantial improvements in employment conditions and immigration policy are germane to their health – matters which are beyond the remit of short-term health promotion projects.

ACKNOWLEDGEMENTS

The author was project manager for SHARP; Helen Thompson was research coordinator; Amin Malik project officer; Dawn Henry and Minara Khatun were research assistants and Lorna McKee was the research consultant. The project was funded as a demonstration project by the Health Education Authority 'Look After Your Heart' programme, as part of the community grant scheme.

NOTE

The views expressed in this chapter are those of the author, and do not represent the views of any other person or the policies of the authorities concerned.

REFERENCES

Adams, L. (1994) 'Health promotion in crisis', *Health Education Journal* 53 (3): 354–60.

Ahmad, W.I.V. (1993) *'Race' and Health in Contemporary Britain*, Buckingham: Open University Press.

Amin, K and Oppenheim, C. (1992) *Poverty in Black and White*, London: Child Poverty Action Group/Runnymede Trust.

Benzeval, M. and Judge, K. (1995) *Tackling Health Inequalities: An Agenda for Action*, London: The King's Fund.

Bhopal, R. (1988) *Setting Priorities for Health Care for Ethnic Minority Groups*, Newcastle upon Tyne: Department of Epidemiology and Public Health, University of Newcastle upon Tyne.

Blakemore, K. and Boneham, M. (1993) *Age, Race and Ethnicity – A Comparative Approach*, Buckingham: Open University Press.

Blaxter, M. (1990) *Health and Lifestyles*, London: Routledge.

Brown, C. (1984) *Black and White Britain: The Third PSI Survey*, Aldershot: Gower.

Department of Health (1992) *The Health of the Nation: A Strategy for Health in England*, London: HMSO.

Douglas, J. (1991) 'Influences on the community development and health movement – a personal view,' in Health Education Unit Open University (ed.) *Roots and Branches: Papers from the Open University Health Education Council Winter School on Community Development and Health*, Milton Keynes: Health Education Unit, The Open University.

—— (1992) 'Black women's health matters: putting Black women on the research agenda', in Roberts, H. (ed.) *Women's Health Matters*, London: Routledge.

—— (1995a) 'Developing anti-racist health promotion strategies', in Bunton, R., Nettleton, S. and Burrows, R. (eds) *The Sociology of Health Promotion*, London: Routledge.

—— (1995b) *Developing Appropriate Research Methodologies for Health and Social Care Research with Black and Minority Ethnic Communities*, Conference Report, West Bromwich: SHARP/Sandwell Health Promotion Unit.

Henry, D., Douglas, J., Thompson, H., Malik, A. and Khatun, M. (1993) *Smethwick – A Community Health Profile*, West Bromwich: SHARP/Sandwell Health Promotion Unit.

Jones, T. (1993) *Britain's Ethnic Minorities*, London: Policy Studies Institute.

Labonte, R. (1993) *Health Promotion and Empowerment: Practice Frameworks*, Toronto: Centre for Health Promotion, University of Toronto.

Lalonde, M. (1975) *A New Perspective on the Health of Canadians*, Ottawa: Information Canada.

MacDonald, G. and Buntin, R. (1992) 'Health promotion – discipline or disciplines?', in Buntin, R. and MacDonald, G. (eds) *Health Promotion – Disciplines and Diversity*, London: Routledge.

McIntyre, S. (1986) 'The patterning of health by social position in contemporary Britain: directions for sociological research', *Social Science and Medicine* 23 (4): 393–415.

Malik, A., Thompson, H., Douglas, J. and McKee, L. (1994) *Smethwick Heart Action Research Project – Developing Heart Health Initiatives with Black and Minority Ethnic Communities*, West Bromwich: SHARP/Sandwell Health Promotion Unit.

Pilgrim, S., Fenton, S., Hugest, T., Hine, C. and Tibbs, N. (1993) *The Bristol Black and Ethnic Minorities Health Survey*, Bristol: University of Bristol.

Rudat, K. (1994) *Health and Lifestyles, Black and Minority Ethnic Groups in England*, London: Health Education Authority.

Smaje, C. (1995) *Health, Race and Ethnicity – Making Sense of the Evidence*, London: King's Fund Institute/SHARE.

Tannahill, A. (1985) 'What is health promotion?', *Health Education Journal* 44 (4): 167–8.

Thompson, H., Douglas, J. and McKee, L. (1993) *Smethwick Heart Action Research Project: Research Process and Methodology*, West Bromwich: SHARP/Sandwell Health Promotion Unit.

—— (1994), *Smethwick Heart Action Research Project, Results of a Health Survey with the African-Caribbean, Bangladeshi, Indian, Pakistani and White Communities in Smethwick*, West Bromwich: SHARP/Sandwell Health Promotion Unit.

Thompson, H., Malik, A., Douglas, J. and McKee, L. (1994b), *Smethwick Heart Action Research Project, Final Report*, West Bromwich: SHARP/ Sandwell Health Promotion Unit.

Tones, B.K. (1983) 'Education and health promotion: new directions', *Journal of the Institute of Health Education* 21: 121–31.

Torkington, P. (1991) *Black Health – A Political Issue*, London: Catholic Association for Racial Justice.

Townsend, P., Whitehead, M. and Davidson, N. (1992) *Inequalities in Health*, London: Penguin.

Whitehead, M. (1989) *Swimming Upstream*, London: King's Fund Institute.

—— (1992) 'The Health Divide', in Townsend, P., Whitehead, M. and Davidson, N. (eds) *Inequalities in Health*, London: Penguin.

Wilkinson, R.G. (1992) 'Income distribution and life expectancy', *British Medical Journal*, 304: 165–8.

Williams, D., Larizzo-Mourney, R. and Warren, R. (1994) 'The concept of race and health status in America', *Public Health Reports* 109 (1): 26–41.

Wilson, M. (1993) *Mental Health and Britain's Black Communities*, London: King's Fund Centre/NHSME Mental Health Task Force/Prince of Wales Advisory Group on Disability.

World Health Organization (1978) *Alma-Ata 1978. Primary Health Care*, Copenhagen: WHO.

—— (1984) *Health Promotion: A Discussion Document on the Concept and Principles*, Copenhagen: WHO.

—— (undated) *Health Promotion – Concept and Principles in Action: A Policy Framework*, Copenhagen: WHO.

—— (1985) *Targets for Health for All*, Copenhagen: WHO.

—— (1986) *Ottawa Charter for Health Promotion*, Ottawa: WHO/Health and Welfare Canada/Canadian Public Health Association.

—— (1988) *The Adelaide Recommendations: Health Public Policy*, Copenhagen: WHO.EURO.

—— (1991) *To Create Supportive Environments for Health. The Sundsvall Handbook*, Geneva: WHO.

Chapter 13

The politics of AIDS treatment information activism

A partisan view

Simon Watney

INTRODUCTION

AIDS treatment activism emerged in the United States (US) in the second half of the 1980s as a response to at least two major factors: the direct experience of acute illness and death presented by the HIV/ AIDS epidemic and a lack of confidence in the capacity or willingness of the medical and pharmaceutical industries to act in the interests of people living with HIV or AIDS. Against a background of profoundly negative social perceptions of the constituencies worst affected by AIDS in the developed world, gay and bisexual men and injecting drug users and their sexual partners, the question of how medical information is generated, by whom and for whom became of major significance for those involved – especially those infected and their immediate friends, families, carers and communities.

This chapter discusses the context in which obtaining and disseminating reliable, up-to-date information in an accessible form emerged as a key issue among AIDS activists and describes and analyses the development of treatment information networks in the wider context of treatment activism, first in the US and subsequently in Britain. The author draws on personal experience and research on both sides of the Atlantic and on recently conducted interviews with key players in establishing and running AIDS information networks in Britain (Edward King, Mark Harrington, Peter Scott and Keith Alcorn). The struggle for a measure of control over information about AIDS and HIV is part of a wider strategy to secure health for individuals, groups and communities which involves a direct challenge to the, at best, benevolent paternalist attitudes of the medical, pharmaceutical and public health establishments and to widespread prejudicial attitudes and behaviours which undermine people's health.

HOW TO MAKE TREATMENT CHOICES IN AN EPIDEMIC

For people living with HIV and AIDS, choices about treatment are bedevilled by the fact that, since the beginning of the AIDS crisis in 1981, rival and incompatible explanations of almost every medical aspect of the epidemic have flourished, from theories concerning modes of transmission and infectivity, to wider questions of the genesis of the epidemic, its extent and the entire field of potential treatments and cures. It remains an interesting question why AIDS has attracted so many 'cranks', conspiracy theorists and anti-rationalists of many different persuasions (Harris 1995). Certainly the situation has not been helped by the generally poor levels of medical journalism throughout the history of the epidemic. In effect, since the isolation of HIV in 1983, the public narratives 'handling' the scientific aspects of AIDS have tended to focus on 'miracle cures' and rivalries between individual scientists, rather than the medical needs of people living with HIV or AIDS.

On the one hand, the mass media has tended to be overwhelmingly fatalistic about AIDS, creating otherwise avoidable stresses for the infected, and on the other hand, the mass media has constantly thrown up seemingly 'scientific' AIDS stories which are frequently unverifiable, or reports of the earliest stages of *in vitro* research. Thus the field of public scientific information on HIV/AIDS has long been muddled with contesting claims. Treatment issues are trivialized as the epidemic itself is sensationalized. All of this is not unconnected to the negative attitudes widely exhibited towards communities most affected by AIDS in the developed world (King 1993; Watney 1994).

These contested claims are frequently presented in the mass media as taking place between 'AIDS heretics' or 'AIDS dissidents' and a supposedly sinister, and complacent 'AIDS establishment' (Harris 1995). However, as Edward King, Editor of *AIDS Treatment Update*, the British monthly AIDS treatment newsletter, has pointed out:

> There really isn't a single 'conventional' view on AIDS for 'dissenters' to disagree with . . . . The vast majority of scientists are convinced that HIV plays a key role in causing AIDS, and that people who are not infected with HIV are not at risk of developing AIDS. However, beyond that there is little consensus. Some researchers think that HIV only causes illness in the presence of other factors. Others think that such co-factors might speed up HIV's harmful effects, but that HIV can still cause illness even in

the absence of co-factors. So here again there is actually a range of opinion, not a party line.

(King 1994)

The use of the term 'AIDS dissidents' suggests the notion of a rigid, conservative orthodox, scientific establishment, challenged like Goliath by plucky, vulnerable, hard-done-by radicals. In practice, however, as King argues:

> the most radical responses to AIDS have come not from AIDS dissidents, but from those working from the inside to challenge the medical model which existed before AIDS. AIDS treatment activism has sought to provide options for people with HIV, and help individuals to make up their own minds about those options. For example, activists have fought to make experimental drugs available as early as possible, through compassionate clinical trial designs and expanded access schemes, so that people with HIV or AIDS at least have the opportunity to take them if they so wish.
>
> (ibid.)

In effect, the many different lobby-groups within the arena of debate about treatment options and research into HIV/AIDS may be roughly divided into those who are, to mimic the language of another controversial health debate, 'pro-choice', and those who are 'anti-choice'. For example, those who proselytize against involvement with what they term 'western medicine', as if it were monolithic, are, in effect, reducing choice for people with HIV or AIDS, just as clearly as those who deny any causal agency between HIV and AIDS provide only the dogmatic assertion that AIDS is somehow caused by the use of recreational drugs or homosexuality and exhibit little or no concern for treatment as an urgent issue for the infected. In reality, surveys clearly demonstrate that most people living with HIV or AIDS use both conventional and complementary medicines, and other therapies, on the basis of informed choices (Barton *et al.* 1994). Such choices are, in any case, often far from easy. For example, whilst one may be looking for beneficial synergistic effects of drugs used in combination, equally it is often the case that different types of drugs which may seem individually advantageous may have harmful consequences when used together. Both the initial need to make choices in the absence of medical understanding of the disease and the subsequent pollution and hijacking of sources of reliable information by lobbies with agendas which precede and exceed HIV/

AIDS, have raised questions about how medical information is produced and disseminated.

THE EMERGENCE OF TREATMENT ACTIVISM

Treatment activism emerged in the US where the epidemic is running approximately five years ahead of the epidemics in Europe. It is also important to recognize that the UK epidemic is disproportionately small by international standards of comparison. Thus, until very recently, Britain has primarily experienced an epidemic of asymptomatic HIV infection, prior to the onset of AIDS, whereas the United States has had a far wider, large scale experience of symptomatic illness and death. By the end of 1994, 260,000 Americans had already died from AIDS (Centre for Disease Control and Prevention 1994), whereas in Britain, with approximately a quarter of the population of the United States, there had been approaching 7,000 deaths (Communicable Disease Surveillance Centre 1994). These figures alone speak of a vastly different social experience of AIDS between cities such as New York and London.

Given this background and the well-known inequalities of American health care provision, it is not surprising that the demand for reliable medical information, couched in practically helpful terms, emerged first in the United States, as increasing numbers of hitherto largely healthy young people sickened and died without effective treatments. Paradoxically, the private, commercial nature of medical provision in the United States had also long encouraged a more generally active role on the part of many patients and patient-groups, in relation to the authority of individual doctors and whole areas of clinical medicine, from paediatrics to oncology. Thus AIDS treatment activism emerged in the mid-1980s in New York and rapidly elsewhere in the United States, within the longstanding American political tradition of voluntary associations, banded together as citizens with specific common goals. Amongst these was a recognition of the need for accessible, reliable, up-to-date information about all and any research that might have some practical therapeutic significance.

A number of community-based periodicals appeared in the mid-1980s in order to 'translate' relevant findings, routinely written up and published in the many different professional scientific journals such as the *British Medical Journal* or *The New England Journal of Medicine*, into pragmatically useful lay terms. The first of these periodicals was *AIDS Treatment News*, which was founded by John S. James in May 1986, initially as a bi-weekly column in the *San Francisco Sentinel*, a local San Francisco gay newspaper. As he explained, back in 1986: '"Beautiful death" ideas were strong in San Francisco, and treatment information was regarded as quackery, false hope which interfered with the process of accepting death' (James 1989: xxix). *AIDS Treatment News* was, and remains, a non-profit organization, with a small staff, and few resources, aiming to: 'contribute to public understanding of how opportunities have been lost in AIDS treatment development, and how past and present problems can be corrected. A humane, informed, and articulate public and professional consensus can save lives' (James 1989: xxxvi).

Very similar motives and aims informed and encouraged the emergence of the AIDS Coalition to Unleash Power (ACT UP) in New York in 1986 (Kramer 1995). However, for ACT UP, treatment information activism was intimately connected to the strategic targeting of institutions understood to be blocking research, or the provision of treatment drugs available in countries such as Britain but unlicensed in the USA. Recognition of the immediately harmful consequences of the market economics of American health care and medical research led initially to the straightforward demand for access to potential treatment drugs, via the provision of more widely available clinical trials. Large numbers of people with HIV had already been recruited into initial clinical trials and the question of the medical ethics of informed consent was widely discussed and written about (Levine *et al.* 1991). Action to secure access to treatment information thus connected closely to campaigns targeting individual pharmaceutical corporations and relevant government departments of the Centers for Disease Control (CDC) and the Food and Drug Administration (FDA), ironically the very departments which had been set up in the 1920s to protect Americans from being exploited, and possibly poisoned, in the search for effective treatments. As playwright Harvey Fierstein explained in a fund-raising letter on behalf of ACT UP in 1988:

> There are times – and I believe this is one of them – when a community has no choice left but to demonstrate to make its voice heard. Quite frankly, I am afraid of what might happen if we don't protest, if we don't take to the streets, if we don't force the government to hear our plea.
>
> (Fierstein 1988)

Hence, in the mid-1980s in the United States, treatment activism involved both the provision of information *and*, frequently, the provision of hard-to-obtain drugs via the appearance of Buyer's Clubs, which varied greatly in the quality of the (often imported) drugs they provided and sold. And from its origins, the People With AIDS Coalition in New York, led by Michael Callen and Michael Hirsch, provided regular treatment data in its publication: the *PWA Newsline*. Only subsequently did the goal of providing treatment information become separate from direct treatment advocacy.

FROM TREATMENT ACTIVISM TO TREATMENT INFORMATION

As ACT UP grew and developed, however, it also became vulnerable to the wider forces of political sectarianism, which saw in AIDS only another example of government neglect or cupidity and recognized no specific medical agenda or priorities. Indeed, as early as Spring 1988, some perceptive AIDS activists were already complaining that:

> Our message is weakened and made partisan when individuals and groups use ACT UP's energy, enthusiasm and demonstrations to promote their non-AIDS political and social agendas regardless of how worthy . . . . Was ACT UP set up to oppose the Reagan administration's foreign policy in Central America? . . . . ACT UP is not affiliated to any political party. When we participate in ACT UP demonstrations we are neither for nor against the Contras, the Sandanistas, the Israelis, the Arabs, nuclear power plants, ICBM's, high tariffs, low tariffs or saving the ozone layer or the dolphins. We are AIDS activists busting our asses to change government policies that are allowing a generation of gay men to die.
>
> (Bramson 1988)

What had been intended as a coalition between the worst affected social communities had become in effect a coalition of left-wing causes. Indeed, by the early 1990s it was frequently argued that the demand for universal socialized medicine in the USA should be the top priority and all questions of HIV/AIDS research should be placed on hold. It was at this point that ACT UP's Treatment and Data Committee resigned and set up their own independent organization, the Treatment Action Group (TAG). Only in this way could expert, pragmatic, achievable demands, which addressed the fact that large numbers of people were dying from AIDS now, be formulated and campaigned for.

Summarizing the current situation in relation to community-based HIV/AIDS US treatment information, leading TAG activist Mark Harrington observes that now:

> most large and many smaller community-based organisations around the country routinely publish treatment updates. Among the most reliable are Gay Men's Health Crisis (GMHC)'s 'Treatment Issues', 'TPA News' from Chicago and 'Critical Path' from Philadelphia. Also of note are local and regional AIDS treatment directories such as AIDS Treatment and Data Network's 'The Experimental Guide' for New York, New Jersey and Connecticut, or the Community Consortium's 'Directory of HIV Clinical Trials in the Bay Area'. The American Foundation For AIDS Research's important and pioneering Directory has now been closed, unfortunately. Niche newsletters include the PWA Health Group's 'Notes From The Underground' and San Francisco's 'Diseased Pariah News' with its important 'Get Fat, Don't Die' column. The New York-based Treatment Action Group (TAG)'s 'TAGline' is also a niche newsletter, in that it focuses on research policy rather than on ground-breaking treatment information per se. In this, and like TAG's periodic reports, it grows from the tradition of activist broadsides, pamphlets and factsheets which were used by ACT UP/ New York in 1988–1992 and particularly its Treatment + Data Committee with a weekly 'T+G Digest' and the annual 'AIDS Treatment Research Agendas'.
>
> (Harrington 1995)

Harrington concludes that many US treatment newsletters have yet to fully come to grips with defining and promulgating standards of what is considered 'reliable' data. Many continue to publish articles based on anecdotes or speculation which, while not necessarily to be excluded, need to be clearly distinguished from the domain of scientific rationality. Noting the continued need for accurate, up-to-date data, Harrington insists that:

> Treatment advocacy needs to continually revisit its original founding principles and see which remain relevant (PWA empowerment and involvement within research, inclusiveness of clinical trials, availability of expanded access programs, continued emphasis on opportunistic infections and cancers) and which need

rethinking (prohibition of placebos, use of clinical endpoints in efficacy trials, criteria for accelerated approval, reliance on surrogate markers, the assumption that a new drug is necessarily better, etc.). Is it possible to ground a vigorous treatment advocacy movement within a framework of realistic (as opposed to Utopian) expectations, and if so, how? There is a lack of historical memory and an insufficient ability to train, mentor and encourage new treatment activists.

(ibid.)

The scale of this task may become more apparent if one considers the sheer volume and complexity of HIV/AIDS research in progress around the world, in need of constant processing and evaluation. For example, the handbook listing papers and poster presentations at the Ninth International AIDS Conference, in Berlin in 1993, came to 672 pages, with an average of some ten different references per page.

The American AIDS information newsletters have now become a central network both for the forging of research and treatment policies and individual decision making – a network which now spills over into E–mail and beyond. Moreover, American models of AIDS activism and advocacy work have been widely influential in other countries with less pronounced and confident traditions of community action coupled to medical scepticism, such as Australia, Canada and the United Kingdom. Yet, of course, the institutions controlling and regulating medical knowledge differ greatly in different countries. Only in a handful of cases has American-style AIDS activism taken root in other parts of the world, such as Paris, where the epidemic is as catastrophic as in most American cities (European Centre For The Epidemiological Monitoring of AIDS 1994) and where the direct effects of illness and death are thus far more widely experienced than in London or Edinburgh. Thus in 'Action': *La Lettre Mensuelle d'ACT UP*, the regular publication of ACT UP/PARIS, treatment information and treatment advocacy remain closely connected behind the slogan *'Info=Vie'* (Information=Life).

TREATMENT INFORMATION ACTIVISM IN BRITAIN

Meanwhile in Britain things are rather different. Writing to complain about a recent article about AIDS in the weekly London listings magazine *Time Out*, a doctor recently invited readers to: 'think about all the politically correct money that has poured into AIDS research at the expense of other diseases. And think about the members of your families who have died, and what killed them?' (Nicholson 1994).

Such attitudes reflect a widespread belief that AIDS research is somehow conducted at the expense of other diseases and medical conditions. Not far behind this lies the less often openly stated belief that people with HIV are not 'like us' (meaning upright heterosexuals) and have only themselves to blame. Indeed, throughout the Thatcher years, the UK mass media and government departments were widely and often persuasively influenced by small, extremist religious and right-wing political groups such as Family and Youth Concern, The Conservative Family Campaign and others (King 1993). In a period of intense competition in the newspaper industry, AIDS has also long been treated as if it were a theoretical issue concerning rival scientific explanations, rather than as an epidemic causing horrific personal and social consequences. Thus the wholly unverifiable assertions of a few individuals and groups with pre-existing moral or political agendas have often been advanced as if they were on the same footing as the consistent research findings of tens of thousands of doctors and researchers around the world (ibid.: Ch. 5). Because there is no baseline to tell us reliably how many gay men there are in the UK it is difficult to assess accurate proportions, but for many years one in four or five gay men attending central London clinics for HIV tests have found they were HIV-positive (King 1993). Moreover the pressures on gay men to take the test are immense. The scale of infection, illness and nowadays death throughout the British gay community, especially in London which has 75 per cent of all UK cases, has no British (or American) parallel in modern times, even in warfare. For example, of the 5,653 deaths from AIDS· up to the end of 1993, 4,291 were amongst gay and bisexual men (Communicable Disease Surveillance Centre 1993). And in recent years, our losses have gone largely unremarked and unlamented, while attention has increasingly focused on 'heterosexual AIDS' (ibid.: Ch.6).

In the early years of the epidemic the British gay press frequently reported news from the US gay press on all aspects of AIDS. Articles from the *New York Native* and *Christopher Street* were summarized within weeks in *Gay News* in London. Yet the number of cases here was small and HIV testing had not yet come into being, so there was little general interest in questions of *cure* compared to the questions of *cause*. As the epidemic unfolded, AIDS Service Organizations emerged from small groups of affected individuals, who recognized clear needs and understood that nobody was going to do anything for the gay community and that we would have to do things for ourselves. Yet groups such as the Terrence Higgins Trust (THT) never regarded the provision of treatment information as being part of their central remit. A group of doctors within the THT simply wrote brief bulletins of the latest information and had no sense of politics around the provision of information. Meanwhile Body Positive, which came into being in 1985, included treatment information in its newsletter, as did several other publications including *Frontliners*, published by and for people with AIDS.

It should also be noted that some small factions of the medical profession and journalists made aggressive attempts to stifle or otherwise invalidate the voices of complementary medicine. This led to a tendency to regard 'official' and complementary medicine as if they were wholly opposed, as if an absolute choice had to be made between the two, rather than choices from *both* options. Similarly, significant legitimate controversy concerning the costs of drugs such as AZT and the possibility of profiteering on the part of the multinational pharmaceutical corporations may also have distracted attention away from the concrete issues of treatment and treatment research goals. Meanwhile, newspapers competed with one another for ever more sensationalist stories about supposedly evil 'AIDS-carriers' and so on. However, some individuals were already connected with the US treatment activism, shipping prescribed drugs for the effective treatment of ailments such as Cyto Megalo Virus retinitis to the United States where they were unavailable and patients simply went blind. Others had close contacts from the beginning with the emergence of ACT UP and reported back to Britain in the gay press.

By the late 1980s it was apparent, however, that Britain was unlikely to see the kinds of pressure that had led to the large scale AIDS treatment activist movement that prevailed in the USA. People would gladly campaign against drug company and health care profiteering but not in favour of particular research, treatment and information policies. This was largely because there were so few people sufficiently on top of the medical literature to be able to formulate an effective critique, if it were needed. There was no UK equivalent to the Treatment and Data Committee of ACT UP in New York and, because of their more deferential relationship with doctors mentioned earlier, British patients tended to expect far less detailed information about their options than Americans.

There was an attempt in the late 1980s to set up a Community Research Initiative (CRI) on New York lines, running clinical trials conducted from GP's surgeries rather than in hospitals, but the competition between the leading London hospitals enforced by government policies undermined the project, since individual hospitals needed to account for patients in order to provide services. Patients could not be 'shared' and GPs were not keen to take on the long-term chronically ill for similar budgetary reasons. In Britain, AIDS activism was honourably concerned with Social Security and housing issues but not with medical policy. As in America, the institutional world of Lesbian and Gay politics, for example, national lobbying groups claiming representational status, seemed (and seem) unwilling to advocate the 'regaying' (King 1993: 169) of HIV/AIDS, usually, it is perversely claimed, 'not to make AIDS look like a gay plague'. Moreover AIDS service organizations, on both sides of the Atlantic, have moved away from a clear identification with the gay (and lesbian) communities from which they first emerged (ibid.: Ch. 5). Thus treatment activists have tended to forge close personal friendships across the Atlantic, rooted in a shared political and ethical perception of the epidemic: what is most urgently needed and how to best achieve such goals.

It was in this context that the *National AIDS Manual* (NAM) was set up by Peter Scott and others in 1988, publishing its first edition in the autumn of that year. NAM came into being as the result of a sense of the general absence in Britain of reliable, up-to-date treatment information, together with accurate data and information on all aspects of the UK epidemic, providing access to further specialist resources and organizations. Most of those at the heart of NAM, including myself, had also had direct experience of the US treatment activist movement, had experienced personal losses early in the epidemic and were long familiar with the various American treatment information newsletters. NAM gained significant help from the American Foundation for AIDS Research (AmFAR), which had begun its far more modest *Treatments Directory* in 1987. NAM was established as an independent, not-for-profit company which could service all HIV/AIDS agencies, having begun as a specialist filing system for London's 24-hour London Lesbian and Gay Switchboard. The aim of NAM was to mediate between the domains of primary research in peer-reviewed medical journals and the type of over-simplified (and often sadly incorrect) data being provided from other sources, especially in relation to treatment options. Funded from sales, together with awards from the Department of Health, pharmaceutical companies, and others, NAM provides an independent voice on HIV/AIDS research.

Scott, the founding Editor of NAM, felt the need to develop a 'learning mechanism' – a form of step-by-step guide to help newcomers understand the issues involved. NAM thus emerged from the self-help model of gay community politics in Britain, with a distrust of the professionalization of AIDS health education and a sense of the publication as a teaching tool, regarding education as a process rather than the provision of, what Scott has described as, 'undigested chunks of raw information' (1995). The strategic intention was that the readership work out for themselves the wider politics revealed by treatment information (for example, about the inequality of access to both clinical trials and treatments between people living in London and those elsewhere).

Initially published in a loose-leaf format, and updating every ninety days, NAM rapidly became the central, reliable text on most specialist aspects of the epidemic in the UK with a current circulation of 1,200 organizations and institutions. Whilst the mass media present AIDS treatment information either sensationally or not at all, NAM continues to provide a balanced centreground between rival and competing extremes. As in America a number of gay doctors played a key role in the provision and checking of information. However, it should be noted that far fewer gay doctors are 'out' at work in Britain than in America, largely because of the more tenacious levels of anti-gay prejudice within the National Health Service and especially amongst consultants who determine medical students' career prospects within the leading medical teaching schools and hospitals in Britain, a topic crying out for detailed research.

NAM is thus a clear example of the type of 'second wave' HIV/AIDS charity, emerging in response to needs that were not apparent to 'first wave' charities, which had never seen the need for treatment information as a high priority. Moreover, treatment information was not regarded as a service they could sell to Local Authority and other financial 'purchasers' within the reorganized economy of British health care provision in the later 1980s and 1990s.

More recently NAM has divided into a series of individual publications, which can be subscribed to separately or together. Thus the NAM *Treatment Directory* specifically covers all aspects of HIV/ AIDS-related medical research, including a detailed survey and analysis of the field of complementary and alternative therapies. NAM has also published a separate AIDS treatment digest, *AIDS Treatment Update* (ATU), on a monthly basis since 1992. This is free for people with HIV or AIDS and is the most widely consulted specialist treatment newsletter in the UK. With a circulation of almost 3,000 individual copies and 600 professional subscribers, ATU aims to provide immediately relevant material for its readership through a combination of general and special issues focusing, for example, on matters of particular relevance to women (for example, Issue 29, May 1995).

It remains to be seen, however, whether the provision of accurate treatment information will eventually translate into treatment activism of the type which in America has so successfully influenced pharmaceutical companies and others. It should be remembered that in the US it was born from a unique sense of emergency, focused largely within a particular social constituency. As yet, in the UK, involvement in HIV/AIDS treatment activism is confined to a small number of people and it is unclear whether or not it might provide a model for other 'disease-communities'. As Edward King, Editor of ATU says:

> ATU aims to provide an environment and, as it were, tools to enable treatment activism to emerge. In the absence of a treatment activist movement in Britain, we wanted to provide a pre-requisite for the emergence of such a movement, based on what is securely known, and most up-to-date. But even after three years there's no indication it has resulted in any more treatment activism in Britain. Perhaps something we did or didn't do caused this. Perhaps people think it's all being done by us for them? Or it may be that activism requires more people with a different personal investment in getting involved?
>
> (1995)

It should also be noted that the domain of AIDS treatment information in the UK remains heavily contested by conflicting and frankly incompatible lobbies. For example, small groups such as Gays Against Genocide (GAG) can relatively easily obtain wide scale press and television coverage for views that are based on the belief that pharmaceutical companies and, in effect, the entire medical profession together with all existing AIDS agencies, are deliberately trying to kill people with poisonous drugs, and that HIV has no role whatever in relation to AIDS or any other aspect of human health (McKerrow and Woods 1993). Picketing organizations such as the Terrence Higgins Trust and publicly branding individual doctors and AIDS workers, including myself, as 'murderers', GAG and others have contributed mightily to spreading confusion, misunderstanding and anxiety amongst people living with HIV and AIDS.

Nor are such diversionary and divisive tactics peculiar to Britain. The author clearly remembers the poignant spectacle of a group of American AIDS workers and activists joining a protest march in Florence at the beginning of the 1992 Seventh International AIDS conference, until it was explained to them that this was a demonstration *against* the provision of needle-exchanges, organized by an Italo-French right-wing New Age group fronted by a charismatic guru, hiding behind a public face of fashionable anti-vivisectionist concern! Such are the contradictions of AIDS treatment information in Europe. Certainly the various bureaucracies of the European Union have been at least as slow as any other major international body to recognize AIDS as a serious crisis or the need for accurate information for the hundreds of thousands of those directly affected throughout the EU, or their communities. It remains to be seen whether or not publications such as *European AIDS Treatment News*, produced by the European AIDS Treatment Group, based in Berlin, will, in time, create a well-informed readership, calmly explaining AIDS for and from the position of the infected, rather than as a confusing and frightening nightmare.

CONCLUSION

Edward King summarizes the major contribution and achievements of AIDS information newsletters and other publications as follows:

> They've been able to get absolutely on top of the material and taken together they give you an amazingly complete picture of the available medical information and debates and choices. In the U.S. these days you have a sort of network of specialist publications, which is a long way from how they all began, when 'AIDS Treatment News' and others were all more or less seen as tools simply to inform people with HIV about current approved and experimental treatment options.

> In the U.K. it is all a lot different, since 'AIDS Treatment Update'

is doing more or less exactly what the U.S. publications were doing some seven years ago. I want ATU material to be as practical as possible. We only very rarely publish anything that doesn't have immediate relevance for people facing treatment decisions in British clinics. The other thing we have been trying to do, in simple terms, is to encourage wider understanding of the complexities of medical treatment issues, whilst at the same time providing straightforward, factual, accessible information. At the same time we go to great pains to highlight the doubts and uncertainties and the conflicts of opinion that characterise much of AIDS research. I think we probably do that better than most other people. Yet many doctors, and others, when they hear the phrase 'treatment activism', probably think of 'GAG' rather than 'NAM' or 'ΛTU'. What a world!

(King 1995)

The history of the provision of community-based HIV/AIDS treatment information and other forms of treatment-based activism suggests a number of initial lessons. First, the process of carefully sifting through and translating vast quantities of highly complex medical data into practical, applicable terms, has already helped transform relationships between doctors and people with HIV and AIDS. Patients are empowered in relation to their primary care providers and others and nobody need today face the frightening uncertainties that prevailed ten years ago.

Second, this history also teaches something of the ways in which treatment issues may be vulnerable to attempted hijacking from either the Left or the Right, who enter the arena with other prior agenda which are usually divisive and distracting from the specific goals motivating community-based treatment specialists. Such would-be 'entryism' is itself perhaps symptomatic of extremist political forces which have few political sites or institutions left open to them in Britain today.

Third, it demonstrates how allopathic and complementary medicine may be regarded and articulated together, from the perspective of potential clients and carers and other service providers, rather than being constantly opposed to one another, with unhelpful degrees of mutual mistrust and hostility.

Fourth, it seems increasingly clear that different national cultural features, as well as local levels of infection, play a significant role in defining and directing different types of treatment advocacy and activism. In Britain, for example, it is probable that there has simply not been the scale of problems harmfully affecting the health of people living with HIV and AIDS, compared to the situation in the United States, for example, or France.

Fifth, and finally, it teaches the need to be able to define achievable aims and appropriate strategies for realizing them. In this respect, as in many others, the movement for greater control over the production and dissemination of HIV/AIDS treatment information may provide a model for other groups of 'patients'. It was thus heartening to recently hear anecdotally that NAM's 1994 *Directory of Complementary and Alternative Therapies* is regarded as indispensable by a group of Scottish cancer patients to whom it was given. It is, of course, primarily for people living with HIV or AIDS to decide on the success or otherwise of our efforts.

REFERENCES

Barton, S., Davies, S., Schroeder, K., Arthur, G. and Gazzard, B.G. (1994) 'Complementary therapies used by people with HIV infection' (letter), AIDS 8: 561.
Bramson, H. (1988) *A Plea For Common Sense*, New York: ACT UP.
Centre For Disease Control and Prevention (1994) *HIV/AIDS Surveillance Report* 6 (2): 19.
Communicable Disease Surveillance Centre (1993) 'AIDS and HIV-1 infections in the UK: monthly report', *Communicable Disease Report*, December: Collingwood.
—— (1994) 'AIDS and HIV-1 infections in the UK: monthly report', *Communicable Disease Report*, December: Collingwood.
European Centre for the Epidemiological Monitoring of AIDS (1994) *AIDS Surveillance in Europe Quarterly Report* 44, December: Brussels.
Fierstein, H. (1988) *ACT UP Fund-raising Letter*, ACT -UP August: 3.
Harrington, M. (1995) personal communication.
Harris, S. B. (1995) 'The AIDS heresies: a case-study in scepticism taken too far', *Sceptic Magazine* 3 (2).
James, S.J.(1989) 'Introduction. Overview: AIDS treatment research and public policy – yesterday and today', in James, S.J. *AIDS Treatment News: Issues 1 through 75, April 1986 through March 1989*, Berkeley CA: Celestial Arts.
King, E. (1993) *Safety in Numbers*, London: Cassell.
—— (1994) 'Out of the margins', *The Pink Paper* 21: 13.
—— (1995) Personal Communication.
Kramer, L. (1995) *Reports from the Holocaust: The Story of an AIDS Activist*, London: Cassell.
Levine, C., Dubbler, N.N. and Levine, R.J. (1991) 'Building a new consensus: ethical principles and policies for clinical research on HIV/

AIDS', *International Research Bulletin: A Review of Human Subjects Research* 13 (1–2): 1–17.

McKerrow, G. and Woods, C. (1993) 'The Angry Young Men of GAG', *Capital Gay* July 16: 16–17.

Nicholson, D. (1994) 'HIV negative', *Time Out* December 7–14: 178.

Scott, P. (1995) Personal Communication.

Watney, S. (1994) *Practices of Freedom: Selected Writings on HIV/AIDS*, London: Rivers Oram Press.

Index